Doping and Anti-Doping in A

This is the first book to focus on the problem of performance-enhancing substances and methods – also known as doping – in sports from African perspectives.

Placing traditional African thinking and indigenous knowledge systems at the centre of the analysis, this book shines new light on the distinctive characteristics of African sporting cultures, doping practices, the management of anti-doping, and new methods for preventing doping in sports that take into account African value systems. This book draws on multidisciplinary work from philosophy, ethics, sociology, history, and political science, and presents real-world case studies of doping and anti-doping from across the African continent. It explores key themes and sites in African sport, culture, and society, including African art, traditional medicine, attitudes towards doping in Africa, sport policy, education systems, media and communications, and the problem of privacy in African sports. This book also considers the uniquely African challenges in anti-doping against the background of the World Anti-Doping Agency policy and practice, and wider international anti-doping efforts.

This book is a fascinating reading for students and researchers with an interest in sport studies, African studies, crime and deviance or public policy, and for sports administrators, sports policymakers, or practitioners working in international, national, or regional sports organisations.

Yamikani Ndasauka is Associate Professor in the Department of Philosophy at the University of Malawi. His research interests are philosophy, applied ethics, and mental health. He is also Editor of the *Journal of Humanities*.

Simon Mathias Makwinja is Senior Lecturer in the Department of Philosophy at the University of Malawi. His research falls broadly within African philosophy. His research interests are in the African thought and value systems.

Routledge Research in Sport, Culture and Society

Sport, Performance and Sustainability
Edited by Daniel Svensson, Erik Backman, Susanna Hedenborg and Sverker Sörlin

The Future of Motorsports
Business, Politics and Society
Edited by Hans Erik Næss and Simon Chadwick

Experiencing the Body in Yoga Practice
Meanings and Knowledge Transfer
Krzysztof T. Konecki, Aleksandra Płaczek, and Dagmara Tarasiuk

Boxing, Narrative and Culture
Critical Perspectives
Edited by Sarah Crews and P. Solomon Lennox

Cricket, Capitalism and Class
From the Village Green to the Cricket Industry
Chris McMillan

Indigenous, Traditional, and Folk Sports
Contesting Modernities
Mariann Vaczi and Alan Bairner

Doping and Anti-Doping in Africa
Theory and Practice
Edited by Yamikani Ndasauka and Simon Mathias Makwinja

For more information about this series, please visit: www.routledge.com/routledgeresearchinsportcultureandsociety/book-series/RRSCS

Doping and Anti-Doping in Africa

Theory and Practice

Edited by Yamikani Ndasauka and Simon Mathias Makwinja

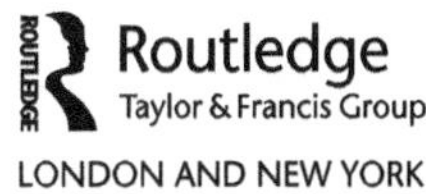

LONDON AND NEW YORK

First published 2024
by Routledge
4 Park Square, Milton Park, Abingdon, Oxon OX14 4RN

and by Routledge
605 Third Avenue, New York, NY 10158

Routledge is an imprint of the Taylor & Francis Group, an informa business

British Library Cataloguing-in-Publication Data
A catalogue record for this book is available from the British Library

ISBN: 978-1-032-44162-7 (hbk)
ISBN: 978-1-032-44165-8 (pbk)
ISBN: 978-1-003-37079-6 (ebk)

DOI: 10.4324/9781003370796

Typeset in Optima
by Newgen Publishing UK

Contents

Acknowledgements

We thank all the contributors for making this work possible. We also thank the World Anti-Doping Agency (WADA) for funding a project (Umunthu and Anti-Doping in Malawi) that inspired this work. Finally, a huge thanks should go to members of the Philosophy Department at the University of Malawi for encouraging us as we undertook this project.

Contributors

Enock Chisati is Associate Professor in the Department of Rehabilitation Sciences at Kamuzu University of Health Sciences (KUHeS), Malawi. His research falls broadly within exercise physiology. He is also interested in sports performance, clean sports, and injury prevention.

Beaton Galafa teaches French in the Department of Language, Linguistics and Classical Studies at the University of Malawi. His research interests include French and Francophone studies, comparative literature, Sino-African studies, and comparative education.

Akuzike Kafwamba is the Country Manager at Business Partners International Malawi. He holds a First-Class Master's Degree in Business Administration from Amity University of India. Akuzike Kafwamba is a Super League of Malawi (SULOM) Executive member. He has also served as a General Secretary for Mighty Tigers Football Club.

Manuel Kasulu is Staff Associate in the Department of Philosophy, University of Malawi. His research explores artificial intelligence (AI) ethics, reality, and subjective experiences. His research interests are ethics of AI, metaphysics, phenomenology, and existentialism.

Maya Kateka is a Sports for Development Associate at the African Union Sports Council Headquarters, Cameroon. Her research interests are sports governance, sports for development, and sports development, especially in Africa.

Blessings Kaunda-Khangamwa is Medical Anthropologist, Public Health Specialist, and Research Consultant at the Kamuzu University of Health Sciences (KUHeS), Malawi. She is an honorary researcher at the University of the Witwatersrand, Johannesburg, South Africa. Her research interest includes medical anthropology, gender, innovative methodological approaches, (non)infectious diseases, adolescent sexuality and reproductive health, and climate change and the environment.

Fiskani Kondowe is Lecturer in the Department of Mathematical Sciences at the University of Malawi. She is also Marie-Curie Early-Stage Researcher at the Centre for Biostatistics at the University of Manchester, UK. Her research interests are statistical methods in child and maternal health, fertility, and mental health.

Jean-Christophe Lapouble is Professor at the University of Poitiers, France, and has been working on doping for more than 30 years. His research focuses, in particular, on fundamental rights in sports and the modernisation of administration, particularly in Africa. He is also a lawyer in Lyon.

Agatha Magombo is Part-time Lecturer in the Department of Philosophy at the University of Malawi. Her research interests lie in ethics and adolescent well-being.

Beullah Matinhira is Lecturer in the Department of Philosophy, Religion and Ethics at the University of Zimbabwe, where she teaches a wide range of philosophy courses at the undergraduate level. She is a registered DPhil candidate with the University of Zimbabwe. Her research interests are in applied ethics.

Tawanda Mbewe is Lecturer at the University of Zimbabwe. He teaches Logic and Ethics. His research interests are in the areas of biomedical ethics as well as gender issues. He is currently pursuing his PhD studies at the University of Zimbabwe.

Frank George Mgungwe is a Development Practitioner and a rural football pundit in Ntchisi, Malawi. His research interests are family law, development, education, and right of the child law.

Stella Patience Mikwana is a Tutor and Researcher in the Department of Philosophy at the University of Malawi. Her main research interests are in applied ethics and African philosophy.

Dave Mankhokwe Namusanya is a PhD candidate at Abertay University, UK. His research interests lie within African indigenous knowledge systems, social justice, and the broader social sciences. His works have been published in various health, communication, criminology, and sociology journals. He has also presented at multiple national and international conferences.

Charles Nyasa is a Registered Physiotherapist and Anatomist, and Lecturer in the Department of Biomedical Sciences at Kamuzu University of Health Sciences (KUHeS), Malawi. Charles is also a Certified Sports Administrator. In 2018, he received the Commonwealth Points of Light Award from Her Majesty Queen Elizabeth II for his work in sports development for people with disabilities.

Mwaona Nyirongo is a PhD student in Journalism and Media Studies at Rhodes University, South Africa. He is also the Executive Director of Malawi China Research Network. His research revolves around sports journalism, public culture, convivial thinking, forced migration, and Malawi China mediascape.

Chapter 1

Introduction to Doping and Sports in Africa

Yamikani Ndasauka and Simon Mathias Makwinja

1.1 Introduction

Sports have been studied from many perspectives, including ethics, health, law, politics, policy, and governance. Each area focuses on a specific dimension of sports. Ethics examines right and wrong in sports. One of delicate ethical issues in sports is cheating, which comes in numerous forms, among them is the use of performance-enhancing substances and methods, known as doping. Doping has become a worldwide problem. Athletes dope to improve their athletic performance, which gives them a competitive advantage over those who do not dope. As a critical problem for sports, doping has been understood and approached from various domains. Some domains that have taken the doping issue seriously include physiology, psychology, ethics, law, culture, medicine, policy, and governance. Arguments that demonstrate the morality or immorality of this practice are commonplace. On account of this, the main objective in all these domains has been to stop doping behaviour and start the practice of clean sports because doping can erode public confidence in sports competitions (Ruwuya et al., 2022, p. 1). However, most existing anti-doping regulations have not been as effective as hoped, or have been effective in a single and small area while the other areas remain unaffected or continue to be the blind spots for any meaningful intervention.

Barrie Houlihan and Dag Vidar Hanstad (2018) assessed the effectiveness of the World Anti-Doping Agency (WADA), the lead organisation in the anti-doping policy and practice. Some of the possible explanations behind the apparent lack of regime effectiveness of WADA included scientific advances in doping, such as "designer drugs", under-resourcing of anti-doping activity in some countries, obstruction in some countries, which include Brazil, Kenya, and Jamaica, and the duplicity of some governments and international federations.

Although doping is a phenomenon that affects sports competitions globally, scholars have observed that African countries face challenges in establishing anti-doping support structures and implementing WADA's anti-doping policy. African countries have limited opportunities to study sports and related areas

DOI: 10.4324/9781003370796-1

in Africa. This has made them develop minimal human resource capacity in sports management. This limited human capacity has negatively affected service delivery in sports and sports development. Besides, the lack of expertise is a massive challenge for anti-doping policy implementation, education programmes, and general sports management. On the academic front, a Western-European perspective has dominated research on anti-doping policy (Ruwuya et al., 2022, pp. 1–3). This could be attributed to how sports are generally conceived in Africa as just pastime with no economic dividends.

However, African countries are increasingly producing elite athletes in many sporting disciplines today. Such athletes are subjected to laws, ethical dilemmas, and anti-doping policies crafted from Western perspectives, even though 47 African countries have ratified the Convention against doping. This ratification requires African national sports organisations to implement anti-doping laws and policies such as whereabouts requirements (Lapouble, 2017, p. 1). These non-African perspectives might not apply to the cultural or ethical life of African athletes. This will make it difficult to understand the anti-doping fight. Although Angella J. Schneider and Theodore Friedmann (2006, p. 1) argue that we can only root out doping behaviour and practices in sports when we understand doping fundamentals, African nations must understand their existential conditions first to develop their own homemade and anti-doping solid structures. Such an understanding is critical for developing robust and effective anti-doping initiatives consistent with their existential needs. This is what the current volume is all about.

Although not exhaustive in examining doping issues, policies, challenges, and opportunities in Africa, the current book is the first to review doping and anti-doping initiatives in Africa. It explores and provokes the doping and anti-doping debate reflecting the unique existential situation of African nations while acknowledging that doping has become a global phenomenon, with noticeable implications in many aspects of human life in general and that of African athletes in particular. One of the central arguments advanced in this book is that doping is not only illegal or dangerous to health as provided for within the Western legal instruments or as proven by Western medical laboratories, but also that doping is essentially a form of cheating one's way to victory. Those familiar with dominant African conceptions of personhood would agree that personhood embodies certain ethical presuppositions (Gyekye, 2011). Such notions of personhood could be handy and explored in developing an educational framework to prevent athletes from using performance-enhancing substances and methods in sports.

1.2 A Glance at the Book

This book is divided into two broader areas: theories and practices surrounding the anti-doping initiatives in Africa. In Chapter 2, Simon Mathias Makwinja and Yamikani Ndasauka discuss how sub-Saharan Africa's

Umunthu ethics or value system can be a framework for anti-doping initiatives in sports. Since the Umunthu philosophy or value system is permeated with principles that guide life among people of sub-Saharan Africa, especially the communitarian ethos, athletes from this region can quickly assimilate it. In Chapter 3, which builds on Jean-Marc Rigaux's 2020 novel, *Kipjiru 42... 195*, Beaton Galafa examines the representation of doping in African athletics. Galafa explains that the novel's theme, plot, characters, and setting revolve around an East African experience of doping in world athletics. In addition, doping in African athletics is regarded in this novel as a regular occurrence orchestrated by highly organised syndicates. Rigaux treats the novel as a window into an African experience of doping scandals, violence, and death.

Chapter 4 by Beullah Matinhira and Tawanda Mbewe advocates for the application of the ethics of Ubuntu/Hunhu, which stresses such values as collectiveness, belonging, and relatedness through its emphasis on humanity, compassion, and social responsibility, as an effective and lasting solution in the fight against doping in sports. In their argument, although Ubuntu/Hunhu is an African moral value system that is in sync with the expectations and worldviews of the African people, it can also be harnessed to suit the global worldview. As an African moral theory, Ubuntu/Hunhu emphasises the importance of collective responsibility over individual preferences. Thus, Ubuntu/Hunhu can be incorporated as a solid pillar to cope with the adverse effects of doping. In Chapter 5, Tawanda Mbewe discusses the sociocultural implications of doping, particularly on the African value system hugely premised on Ubuntu. The moral values of Ubuntu have not been spared the threat of doping activities.

In Chapter 6, Stella Mikwana, Agatha Magombo, Manuel Kasulu, and Yamikani Ndasauka explore the use of African indigenous remedies and rituals in sports, especially how they satisfy the criteria for doping as ascribed by WADA. They also explore the perceived effectiveness of the said remedies and ritual practices, propose revising WADA's criteria, and find other ways to regulate or prohibit traditional sports remedies. This is in response to the growing need for WADA to redefine doping standards. They argue that some practices in African indigenous knowledge systems in sports embody doping parameters. In Chapter 7, Jean-Christophe Lapouble argues that the World Anti-Doping Code is mainly theoretical in Africa. Indeed, if most African countries adhere to the system set up by WADA, very few can apply it effectively. The numerous difficulties that African countries may experience due to their degraded socio-economic context confine anti-doping policies to the rank of non-priority public policies. In general, the challenges experienced by different countries in terms of development, structuring of the sports movement through associations, public administration, public health, and corruption provide sufficient evidence to argue that the fight against doping in Africa cannot be free from the socio-economic context and must therefore be adapted accordingly.

Chapter 8 by Mwaona Nyirongo explores how anti-doping news is presented in Malawian sports news, especially in the *Daily Times* and the *Nation*. The resort to the newspapers is because of the unavailability of adequate studies that conceptualise doping from an African perspective. Thus, from these newspapers, Nyirongo identified anti-doping themes that journalists want their audience to think about, how to think about them, and how to sustain such thoughts. The chapter establishes that anti-doping news mostly frames athletic bodies as childish and crooked, while the country's legal structures are perceived as inadequate. Chapter 9 by Charles Nyasa, Blessings Kaunda, and Enock Chisati reviews the component functions of the World Anti-Doping Programme and discusses levels of their implementation at national level sports. The discussion takes Malawi as a point of reference due to its underdeveloped sports systems, scanty literature, and a culturally pinned drug use context that closely characterise most non-Western resource-limited nations.

In Chapter 10, Frank Mgungwe exposes retrogressive practices in rural communities by juxtaposing instances which reflect convincingly effective "witchcraft doping" with instances that reflect an apparent failure of attempted "witchcraft doping". In Mgungwe's argument, "witchcraft doping" creates a false-positive illusion of effectiveness among competitors, affecting or influencing their on-the-pitch performance like in the placebo effect. Rumours, speculations, and accusations of "witchcraft doping", characterising event build-up conversations, are an obvious recipe for conflicts, fights, and pitch invasions if unusual misses, misfiring, and poor officiation occur. Chapter 11 by Beullah Matinhira discusses the role played by a combination of environmental factors leading to the use of performance-enhancing drugs in Africa. The assumption is that doping is a socially complex problem, not just an individual choice. For example, the existence of competitive pressure and the pursuit of victory in the world of sports provide a fertile ground for doping behaviour to take place. In Africa, values such as reciprocity, communality, interrelatedness, and interconnectedness, among others, could contribute to the "dopogenic" space. In Chapter 12, Dave Namusanya argues that sports doping in Africa wears a different face whose understanding transcends the mainstream version of the practice. To do so, he uses the ecologies of knowledge approach to argue for the need to reconceptualise doping practice within the public imaginary while highlighting the perversity of *Juju* narratives in the African and Malawian public spaces.

In Chapter 13, Manuel Kasulu, Stella Mikwana, Agatha Magombo, and Yamikani Ndasauka present an argument that WADA's whereabouts requirements for anti-doping are inconsistent with the sociocultural context of African athletes and the two-dimensional conception of time that is predominant among Africans. Since African athletes live in predominantly communitarian societies with numerous obligations to their communities and immediate families, these anti-doping obligations make it difficult to abide by WADA's whereabouts requirements. The authors propose a reconstruction of WADA's whereabouts requirements established on the principles of trust and individual liberty. They hope that the proposed reconstruction of WADA's whereabouts requirements will simultaneously promote the sociocultural well-being of African athletes and WADA's objective to eliminate out-of-competition doping. Chapter 14 by Yamikani Ndasauka, Maya Kateka, Fiskani Kondowe, Simon Makwinja, and Akuzike Kafwamba assesses the gaps in anti-doping initiatives in Malawi. Specifically, it engages athletes' rating of the athlete support personnel's (ASP) role as a source of trusted information on anti-doping. It further asks whether the ASP themselves understand their respective roles in anti-doping.

1.3 Conclusion

When the readers pass through these chapters, we hope to ignite their intellectual curiosity regarding doping and the various anti-doping initiatives. Above all, we hope that this book would inspire many to join the doping and anti-doping dialogue with its multifaceted dimensions. Our desire is for scholars, athletes, sports organisers, administrators, as well as spectators involved in various sporting disciplines to now see the sense of urgency surrounding sports doping and that anti-doping initiatives require the participation and contribution of all. The ultimate aim is to promote clean sports.

References

Gyekye, K. (2011). African ethics. *The Stanford Encyclopedia of Philosophy* (Fall 2011 Edition), Edward N. Zalta (ed.). Available at https://plato.stanford.edu/archives/fall2011/entries/african-ethics/

Houlihan, B., and Hanstad, D.V. (2018). The effectiveness of the World Anti-Doping Agency: developing a framework for analysis. *International Journal of Sport Policy and Politics, 11*(2), 203–217. https://doi.org/10.1080/19406940.2018.1534257

Lapouble, J.-C. (2017). Athlete whereabouts in the context of the fight against doping in Africa; mission impossible? *African Sports Law and Business Bulletin, 1*, 1–7.

Ruwuya, J., Juma, B.O., and Woolf, J. (2022). Challenges associated with implementing anti-doping policy and programs in Africa. *Frontiers in Sports and Active Living, 4*, 1–7. https://doi.org/10.3389/fspor.2022.966559

Schneider, A.J., and Friedmann, T. (2006). The problem of doping in sports. In J.C. Hall, J.C. Dunlap, T. Friedmann, and V. van Heyningen (Eds.), *Advances in Genetics: Volume 51. Gene Doping in Sports: The Science and Ethics of Genetically Modified Athletes*. Cambridge, MA: Academic Press (pp. 1–9). https://doi.org/10.1016/S0065-2660(06)51001-6

Part I

African Thought and Doping

Chapter 2

Umunthu Ethics as a Framework for Anti-Doping Education

Simon Mathias Makwinja and Yamikani Ndasauka

2.1 Introduction

The sporting universe faces several challenges, such as violence (both on and off the pitch), hooliganism, discrimination, racism, doping, match-fixing, corruption, and vandalism. One of the most critical and exciting challenges is using performance-enhancing substances and methods, technically called doping. Societies worldwide have generally accepted that doping is a form of manipulation of sports. Such a manipulation which alters performance and its results is undesirable. As such, this challenge requires deliberate control, regulation, and even banning since it is against what is perceived as the standard way of participating in sports. In other words, doping results in a manipulated, mediated, or unnatural success.

Schneider and Friedmann (2006) have suggested banning doping or other sports manipulation to achieve athletic excellence. The justification for prohibiting doping includes the consideration that doping in sports is essentially a form of cheating and, therefore, unfair; doping in sports harms athletes; doping harms even non-doping athletes in the sense that those who compete without doping are put under immense pressure; doping damages society, especially children who see athletes as role models; testing and monitoring to detect instances of the illicit drug is very expensive; doping represents a perverse behaviour in sports; and that doping is unnatural and dehumanising.

Given the dangers posed by doping, the continued involvement of athletes in doping, and the complications and costs involved in testing to take appropriate action against those involved in this illegal, unethical, and wrong sports practice, there is a need for "new approaches developed from 'out-of-the-box' thinking" such as the involvement of sports physicians in the fight against doping (Dvorak et al., 2014, p. 3). But, as they say, a stitch in time saves nine, or prevention is better than cure, better complementary approaches to doping would be those that prevent athletes from even attempting an illegal or unethical manipulation of sports results. Such approaches would be the cheapest, with limited intrusion into athletes' private lives. For this reason, the 2015

DOI: 10.4324/9781003370796-3

World Anti-Doping Code focuses on preventing doping through education programmes across different age groups and sporting disciplines.

Not every educational framework works for every athlete, owing to their differences in cultures and value systems. A practical educational framework must be culturally relevant and one that athletes must easily relate to and ultimately internalise in their daily endeavours. Culture provides individuals with definite patterns of behaviour and values which guide their conduct. According to Gamage et al. (2021, p. 1), values are the inner realities of an individual that are reflected through habits, behaviours, beliefs, expectations, and relationships. In this regard, this chapter proposes using the Umunthu philosophy or value system to prevent doping among athletes, especially athletes from the sub-Saharan region. Umunthu is regarded as a philosophy or value system that guides everyday activities and behaviour among peoples of sub-Saharan Africa. The assumption is that athletes from the sub-Saharan region can easily relate to this value system. As a way of life and a value system, Umunthu is imbued with elements vital for the proper functioning of the individual in relation to the community.

In its attempt to show how Umunthu philosophy or value system can help to prevent athletes from actually involving themselves in sports doping, the chapter has six small sections. The following sections discuss doping prevention in sports and priority areas of anti-doping activities. Then the nature of sports through human nature will be addressed. This will be followed by demonstrating why doping in sports is unethical. Then the chapter will briefly engage the Umunthu philosophy or value system. Finally, there will be a demonstration of how Umunthu values can prevent doping behaviour among athletes, thereby significantly contributing to anti-doping initiatives.

2.2 Prevention of Doping in Sports

Doping in sports today does not only affect the athletes psychologically like it was assumed in the past. The drugs which athletes currently use are also hazardous. They have the potential of not only having powerful and real effects on athletic performance which is primarily sought, but also equally harming the athletes psychologically (Schneider and Friedmann, 2006). In addition, doping has not only become more diverse, highly specialised, and efficient, but above all, it is also dangerous for the health of athletes (Peskov, 2019). For this reason, specific organisations have been tasked with the responsibility to fight the prevalence of doping. On account of the dangers associated with many forms of doping, there have been regulatory mechanisms to help detect and control drug-based doping in sports. Hence, the International Olympic Committee (IOC) has for a long time attempted to stop this problem, but with little success.

Nowadays, corruption has been identified as one of those factors that help athletes to escape the responsibility of doping, especially through the granting of exceptions on therapeutic use of drugs (see Peskov, 2019). In addition, there are many new, more powerful, and undetectable doping techniques and substances which are now abused by professional athletes. Furthermore, now there exist sophisticated networks of illicit drugs distribution (Baron et al., 2007, p. 118). Schneider and Friedmann (2006, p. 7) suggest that if athletes and their managers are given an opportunity, they are likely to exploit it and use the many illicit techniques and substances to provide them with a competitive advantage over others in sports. Indeed, modern sport does not only offer entertainment and prestige to participants and their nations or clubs or associations, but also turns out to be a huge business involving insane amounts of money.

Since sport has become an industry or a business in the contemporary world, chances are high for individuals to break the rules just to win. Athletes are driven by the desire to compete, excel, and win, even at the cost of injury and other harms to themselves and society. They are ready to take risk including doping just to ensure the victories. Sometimes this is done consciously and camouflaged with a network of specialists behind or on their own. Given that sports involve sponsors, advertising contracts, and money, some athletes believe that any risk is worth taking. As we have said before, some of these risks affect athletes' own health (often with huge and irreversible consequences). Owing to its popularity, sport has been used to promote peace globally.in the world (see Boyacıoğlu and Oğuz, 2016). It is not surprising therefore that sporting events have become some of the most powerful instruments for international politics.

The sole responsibility to lead the fight against doping in sports lies with the World Anti-Doping Agency (WADA) which was formed in 1999. WADA's mission is to work independently of the IOC, sports organisations, and governments to lead the fight against doping in sport. Specifically, WADA is mandated with the development of programmes for detection and control of doping in sports. Thus, it would go on to "harmonise the fight against doping in different sports, coordinate anti-doping activities and create a clearing-house for the management of positive cases" (Dvorak et al., 2014, p. 1). WADA has for a long time prioritised testing and supportive medical treatment which have been regarded as effective in reducing and even stopping doping behaviour. WADA also compiles and constantly updates a list of substances and methods that are inconsistent with sports ideals and that should be banned from competitions (Schneider and Friedmann, 2006, pp. 7–8).

In spite of this systematic, scientific, and aggressive approach to anti-doping testing by WADA and various other international sports federations for sporting disciplines such as cycling, athletics, and soccer, substance abuse scandals involving high-profile athletes have been on the rise across the globe. A number of sporting professionals have been disqualified and even banned from participating in their respective sporting disciplines. For example, the

American athlete Marion Jones, who won three gold medals and two bronze medals at the Sydney Olympics in the year 2000, admitted lying to federal agents about her use of performance-enhancing drugs. She eventually served a six-month jail sentence and had all her five medals stripped by the IOC. Moreover, as Jiri Dvorak et al. (2014, p. 2) concur, WADA's increase in both in and out of competition testing does not prevent an unknown number of athletes from taking performance-enhancing drugs prior to and/or during major competitions.

2.3 Priority Areas in Anti-Doping Activities

Acknowledging the unethical behaviour of doping in sports, and especially the harm it can cause to oneself and society, WADA has been given the unconditional mandate to protect athletes' right to participate in drug-free sport. Specifically, WADA's mandate is to harmonise, coordinate, and carry out effective anti-doping programmes, and focusing on detection, deterrence, and prevention of doping (Gatterer et al., 2020, p. 228).

Gatterer et al. (2020, p. 229) have isolated two priority areas in anti-doping initiatives: deterrence and prevention. Deterrence involves doping testing and exclusion of doping offenders from sport. Prevention consists of provision of information and education. Although there is tremendous increase and improvement in testing techniques, the number of positive test results so far remains low. It is however suggested that the true prevalence numbers are higher. Because of limitations of detection-based deterrence such as the unequal implementation of testing in different sporting disciplines and countries, and limited deterrence effect of testing, emphasis has been placed on the need to give a higher priority to doping prevention-orientated strategies. However, Gatterer et al. (2020, p. 229) report that currently there is a limited amount of research focusing on doping information and education-based prevention activities in different countries. Focus on protective factors should help athletes resist doping even though they are exposed to risk factors that might promote doping behaviour. Ideally, prevention measures decrease the risk of doping and increase protection from doping. In the context of protecting athletes from violating doping rules, personal factors such as strong morality, self-control, and resilience against peer pressure seem to be important.

While education programmes have been proposed as an intervention in the prevention of doping behaviour, not all education programmes are suitable for all people characterised by their belonging to unique cultures and value systems. That is, the same education cannot be successfully applied to all countries and expect the same results. There certainly must be some kind of variations. For this reason, different theoretical perspectives are needed for this objective. By extension, it is the reason this chapter attempts to demonstrate how Umunthu philosophy or value system can become the basis of an education framework that would help athletes avoid doping. It is the opinion of this chapter that although Umunthu philosophy is African, its relevance could go beyond assisting African athletes to become applicable to athletes from other parts of the world in the prevention of doping.

2.4 The Nature of Sports through Human Nature

In modern-day sports, doping has become a very complex issue. The doping phenomenon in sports is increasing and diversifying, as are the drugs and methods. There is a constant and fierce competition between those who invent new doping methods and sports ethics organisations that are searching for more performant methods to detect them. Sports ethics organisations are always looking for improved scientific procedures for detecting prohibited substances. Usually, they involve various levels of authorities to prevent the spread, marketing, and use of such substances.

Cases of doping are said to have compromised the credibility of performance and results in sports. This renders sports methods and results illegal, unethical, and, above all, bad. What makes doping illegal, unethical, and bad is said to be the unnaturalness of the performance-enhancing substances. However, the so-called mediatised victories or unnatural successes (allowing them to retain titles) of some sports heroes become questionable and disputable. But, how does the improvement of human nature with the aim of individual and sometimes collective health (i.e., therapy) become an illegitimate goal in sports and a legitimate one in the treatment of known illnesses?

To meaningfully confront the illegality, unnaturalness, or immorality of doping, there is a need to understand the nature of sports as well as human nature whether they contradict or complement each other. It is not enough to know and communicate about the rules that prohibit certain things in sports, but also the essence of sport itself. Indeed, as Arthur L. Caplan and Brendan Parent (2017, p. 1) argue, "to know what ought to happen and what ought to be prevented in and around sport — the ethics of sport — we should know not only the rules but also the essence of sport". Sport is sometimes played for fun, and often competitively, with players trying their hardest to win games by defeating their opponents. Some people think there is a thin line between sports as a recreational activity and as competitive athletics, although it is largely doubtful that a demarcation exists. What is commonly noticed is a continuum from friendly or amateur games towards those that are more professional.

A meaningful discussion of ethics in sports requires one to consider the level or degree of competitiveness of games. Some critics of competitive sports think that emphasis on competition and winning is ethically indefensible. Others think that the main problem in every competitive sport is the emphasis on competition and winning. Competition and winning, the ugly side of being human, is frequently on display (Aicinena, 2010, p. 15). This position has its justification in Hobbes' hypothetical state of human nature where human beings as eternally in a state of unrestricted competition or conflict. For Hobbes, this state of nature forms the basis and defence of his postulations on the need for law and order. Life without law and order would be bleak and undesirable. In the state of nature there is no law or rule to be enforced on people. Individuals would do anything to secure material resources to survive. In the absence of law and order, any alliances would be based on mutual advantage and would last only so long as it would be in the parties' interest to keep them.

In Hobbes' state of nature, individuals tend to think of their own self-interest first, and place a great emphasis on competitive victory over others. Such individuals focus less on the humanity of others. They consider the status of others as obstacles standing in the way of securing their personal goals. As Charles E. Merriam (1906, p. 151) explains, "there are three principal causes of quarrel among men; first, the desire for gain; second, for safety, and third, for glory". This has led people into the condition of "war". Hence, it is not a far-fetched opinion that competitive sports reflect Hobbesian assumptions about human psychology and state of nature, especially displayed in the intense pursuit of victory and glory. This inevitably leads competitors to view opponents not as persons just like themselves, but as obstacles standing in their way of success. Founded on the philosophy of individualism, sport is understood as an individual activity emphasising individual values and success. As Robert Simon (2016, p. 31) contends, individual athletes tend to think that pursuing personal interest is the highest and perhaps the only legitimate goal they must achieve. Athletes put great weight on competitive victory over others and pay little attention to the humanity of others. In fact, others are seen as obstacles in the way of achieving their personal goals. It is on this basis that one can argue that competitive athletics breeds hostility, enmity, and even hatred of opponents. Through emphasis on competition, some critics accuse sports of promoting selfishness. In the words of Pisk (2011, p. 59), sports consist of "end-directed physical activities, e.g. sport for money, sport for education, sport for health, sport for loss of body weight".

What about spectators' perceptions of the winning or losing athletes?

Sports can also be used to sharpen one's skill in something such as improving one's cognitive abilities in cancer patients (Sebri et al., 2019). Sport should also test natural talent and dedication of competing athletes. As Andrew Bloodworth (2018) argues, sports concern the human natural abilities and efforts to either overcome human physical limitations or to supplement those physical endowments that many elite athletes appear to have. The losers in a sporting competition have something to be proud of as well. In many sporting disciplines, it is customary for winners to show respect to the losers. This act of kindness conveys athletes' trust, balance, acceptance, and respect they have for each other. Despite the aggressive nature of competition for medals, athletes realise that they are simply human. It is from this kind of thinking and doing that an argument can be raised that competitions of all sorts do not always, and perhaps do not usually, embody the disrespect and dehumanisation of the opponent, as some critics fear (Fouché, 2012). For example, Emanuele Isidoria and Mirca Benetton (2015, p. 688) have argued that understanding sports in a commodified way tends to undermine human dignity in many ways. They think that sports can actually develop as a dehumanising practice when they become part of a business society. Players are exploited for various advertising purposes. Players are reduced to objects or things when they are bought and sold. When teams lose, spectators insult players. Besides, as sport is increasingly big business, and crucially associated with big business, it creates opportunity and motivation for corrupt practices (Ibrahim, 2016, p. 67). To a certain extent, and on the basis of such experiences and observations, one can argue about loss of integrity in sports, and that sports dehumanise players since their dignity as human beings is compromised by the sole focus on the results, especially positive results.

Now, the ethical question concerns how sports should be conducted in order to be morally defensible, and to show that sports do not necessarily embody the Hobbesian perspective of human nature. That is, beyond the goal of winning, sports foster other positive human values. Sports provide individuals with a test through the challenge of competition as structured by the established rules and regulations of the sport. In this way, sporting opponents facilitate each other's goal of being tested and are in an at least partially cooperative as well as competitive relationship. Even if it is admitted that human beings are characteristically selfish in the Hobbesian sense, so that their ultimate goal is winning regardless of the circumstances, egoistic tendencies must be kept in constant check if positive human values are to be fostered. Even if rivalry is emphasised in principle, it is common to see mutual respect being encouraged and emphasised in practice. Health and controlled rivalries exist everywhere: academia, business, science, arts, as well as sports. In this regard, sports have the potential to benefit human nature as opposed to the emphasis laid on its ugly side (Simon, 2016).

Within the sporting universe, sporting integrity appears to be a value that is rarely commented upon unless it is noticeably absent. To appreciate the role of ethics and integrity in sports in general, there is a need to explore the distinction people make between gamesmanship and sportsmanship. Gamesmanship and sportsmanship are concepts which embody the progress that sports have made. That is, the progress is from conceiving sports around the Hobbesian sense of human nature whose ultimate goal is winning regardless of the circumstances, exhibiting greater skill and deftness than one's opponent, towards the kind of sports which emphasise improving athletes' character and moral development. Ultimately, this progress deals with negative behaviours of some athletes and coaches. Gamesmanship is built on the sole principle of winning. Within this dimension, athletes and coaches are motivated by egoistic orientation which is often associated with unsportsmanlike attitudes, such as cheating and using deception to gain an advantage over others (Stewart, 2014, p. 5). Players and coaches are encouraged to bend the rules wherever possible in order to gain competitive advantage over an opponent. Through this behaviour, players pay less attention to the safety and welfare of others and of the competition itself because for them, the end always justifies the means. By emphasising winning at all costs, players in many sporting disciplines have feigned injuries; players and coaches have tampered with equipment; players have used performance-enhancing drugs, taunted and intimidated an opponent; coaches have lied about an athlete's age in order to keep him or her eligible to play. All these originate from the great emphasis laid on always winning.

There have been high-profile cases around the question of integrity involving athletes in various sporting disciplines. Consider the famous Lance Armstrong, cycling the Tour de France, who revealed to have actually used performance-enhancing drugs. This is something which he had denied for years. There have been similar cases in cricket and soccer. The fundamental claim which is made, and is said to mirror these incidents, is that the integrity of the sport was damaged. Hence, in recent times, because of overemphasising gamesmanship in almost every sporting discipline, fans, pundits, coaches, and players alike appear to be appealing to the idea of "sporting integrity" when they voice their approval or disapproval of some aspects of behaviours that characterise the sporting activities. In football (soccer), for example, players who dive into the penalty area in order to win a penalty kick are shown a yellow card as a warning for trying to con match officials. If referees went on to award a penalty, they would bring the game into disrepute.

Sportsmanship model of sports on the other hand is built on the idea that sport both demonstrates and encourages character development, which then influences the broader community. The way individuals or teams compete in sports can have an effect on personal moral and ethical behaviour outside of the competition. For this reason, sportsmanship has become an ethical approach to sports, healthy and responsible competition. Sportsmanship is seen as a means of cultivating personal honour, virtue, and character. Sportsmanship contributes to a community of respect and trust between competitors and society. The goal of sportsmanship in sports competitions is not simply about winning while others lose, but also importantly to pursue victory with honour by giving one's best effort. In addition, Alfred Archer (2016, p. 128) has argued that sporting integrity should be viewed as a virtue possessed by sports rather than by sporting competitors or institutions that run it. However, today integrity is expected even from the competitors and institutions because their actions and decisions affect the integrity of sports. It is up to both competitors and institutions to ensure that the integrity of sport is preserved. In this regard, C. Craig Stewart (2014, p. 6) has argued that sportsmanship remains an essential component for the future of sport. Accordingly, this can be seen in the way sport administrators and parents of future athletes continue to show their desire that coaches exhibit and require sportsmanship. Accordingly, it can be argued that sportsmanship provides the humanising elements in sports. From the consideration of the two perspectives of sports, it becomes fairly easy to see the role of ethics in making sports competitions more humane.

2.5 Why Is Doping in Sports Unethical?

All the concerted efforts towards the fight against doping through various policies and regulations assume that doping in sports is unethical, although the least emphasised assumption borders on health. The intention in this section is to demonstrate the said unethicality of doping in sports. We maintain that without coming to grips with what makes doping unethical, all efforts aimed at outlawing it will be useless. In addition, without this demonstration, the proposal to use some elements of the Umunthu value system in dealing with the problem of doping in sports, albeit the fact that there are many other unethical issues in sports, will not make sense. Oftentimes, doping and other unethical behaviours in sports such as match-fixing, corruption, vandalism, hooliganism, violence, and bullying are considered as depriving sports of integrity. Accordingly, these instances result from overemphasis on:

> winning, seeking prestige or financial rewards, bending the rules, cheating, coach aggression, disrespect, and player aggression; [....] verbal abuse, negative coaching behaviors and practices, athletes being pushed too hard by coaches or parents, negative administrative behaviors and practices and negative officiating behaviors and practices.
>
> (Ibrahim, 2016, p. 67)

But what makes such behaviours in sports unethical, bad, and undesirable to the extent of making them unlawful? According to WADA, the organisation mandated to control doping in all sporting disciplines, sports have an intrinsic value. This is the celebration of the human spirit, body and mind, which is reflected in values that are emphasised in sports. These values include fair play and honesty, respect for self and other participants, respect for rules and laws, and health (WADA, 2017, p. 1). WADA has stated three reasons for prohibiting doping, namely, to protect athletes' health, to promote fairness, and to preserve meanings and values in sport. However, as Murray (2017) argues, "the fundamental justification for anti-doping is found in the meanings and values we pursue in and through sport" (p. 186). According to Palmi et al. (2019, p. 1), "unlawful substance abuse is in fact liable to undermine the very core of fairness in competition". The use of substances or methods that enhance athletic performance violates the principles of equal opportunity and fairness between athletes. Those athletes using performance-enhancing substances have competitive advantage over those who simply rely on their naturally endowed abilities. Similarly, Andrew J. Bloodworth and Mike McNamee (2017) also explain that:

> sports can be understood as a means of testing the natural physical abilities of the athlete, combined with the hard work they put into improving their performance. Permitting certain forms of performance enhancement would threaten the special nature of such a test. Doping can be seen as a threat to the integrity of sport, not just because of the rule breaking doping currently entails.
>
> (p. 177)

For the reasons cited above, doping should in fact be regarded as cheating for it does not follow the established rules, although some have argued that doping can actually be morally justified in the way civil disobedience is justified against institutionalised rules (see Vorstenbosch, 2010, p. 167 ff.). In this case, doping is an infidelity. Above all, it leads to unfairness in sports competition, and at the same time causes harm to the society, especially to children and young adults who consider athletes as their role models.

2.6 The Umunthu Philosophy or Value System

In order to demonstrate the potential role that the Umunthu philosophy or value system can play in the reduction of doping in sports, there is a need to consider what Umunthu philosophy or value system actually is. As a CiNyanja term, Umunthu depicts the quality of being human. As a cognate of the popular Ubuntu, which is a pan-African philosophical concept, Umunthu is sometimes simply translated as humanness. The term thus signifies an indigenous philosophy associated with the people of Malawi and neighbouring countries such as Zambia and Mozambique. Umunthu can be expressed as a value system operating across much of sub-Saharan Africa as well as a normative philosophy of how people should relate to one another (Wright and Jayawickrama, 2021, p. 618). Some of Umunthu values are considered as capable of complementing and shaping the direction of anti-doping initiatives. The argument here is that the philosophy of Umunthu can be a pragmatic as well as a proactive approach to the prevention of doping among athletes. Specifically, Umunthu re-enacts respect among athletes who ordinarily compete as opponents.

Umunthu philosophy has been popularised by the cognate concept of Ubuntu. Whatever is said of Ubuntu, the same is entirely applicable to Umunthu. A lot of scholars have commented on the concept and the meaning of Ubuntu. As such, we do not think we are in a position to say anything new or special about the concept and the philosophy of Ubuntu. However, as a number of scholars have done, it is important to re-emphasise that the term "Ubuntu" has its roots in Nguni (isiZulu), especially its maxim: *Umuntu Ngumuntu Ngabantu*, translated as "a person is a person because of or through others" (Chigangaidze and Chinyenze, 2022, p. 280). In African cultures, Ubuntu can be used to describe the capacity for one or a group to express compassion, reciprocity, dignity, solidarity, harmony, consensus, hospitality, sympathy, humanity, mutuality, and sharing among other qualities or values. These values are regarded as central in the building and maintenance of communities characterised by justice and mutual caring (see Chingaidze et al., 2022, p. 319; Wright and Jayawickrama, 2021 p. 618 citing Tutu, 2004, pp. 25–26). Ubuntu is therefore a philosophy, a tradition, or a worldview of people of Southern Africa, having its own distinctive features and method of how one should conduct himself or herself in the public domain. Within Ubuntu, one sees herself or himself as an individual through the existence of others with whom they share the social space. Emphasising on the moral attributes of a person, then, to be human is to establish respectful human relations with others. The philosopher Munyaradzi F. Murove (2012, p. 37) has argued that as a relational being, to be a human being in the Ubuntu way poses a great challenge and a robust alternative to the contemporary individualistic and self-interested understanding of a person. Accordingly, humanness is the existential precondition of one's bondedness with others.

The value of interpersonal relations is emphasised in Ubuntu. Ubuntu conceives of humanity not solely in terms of the individual but also as a collective. Ubuntu stresses the collective success of a group or society. For example, when someone has done something good, the community as a collective also becomes good, and the opposite is true. Through the collective, individuals create and sustain each other through such qualities or values as unity, helpfulness, caring, trust, and respect. These and many others form the essence of Ubuntu. For many scholars Ubuntu philosophy provides a framework for many positive things. It is not surprising therefore that the main objective in this chapter is to apply some of these positive qualities or values to demonstrate their effectiveness in the anti-doping initiatives. It is to this demonstration that we now turn.

2.7 Umunthu Values and Anti-Doping Initiatives

This section isolates some Umunthu values for the purpose of showing the role that this philosophy can play in anti-doping initiatives. Specifically, we are talking of values that can act as a compass to guide activities within the sporting world in avoiding doping. We are aware that it is not all Umunthu values that appear to encourage or build desirable human qualities. Certainly, there exist some values which lack the qualities that would prevent doping in sports. However, we target positive Umunthu values.

One obvious positive value that Umunthu reinforces is the interconnectedness or interdependence of members of a group or community in order for individuals to flourish. In fact, the Umunthu philosophy can only be operationalised through relationships. The essence of the community is for individuals to relate well (Wright and Jayawickrama, 2021, p. 619). The sporting world is a large community. Thus, in the sports domain, interconnectedness or interdependence of members can be exploited to help athletes avoid doping. Athletes will be reminded that their worth or value is inherently tied or connected to the value or humanity of others. Importantly, athletes will consistently be reminded of the primacy of humanity of their fellow competitors. If one recognises that she has more similarities than differences with her competitor, she is likely to respect them or in this case show them Umunthu. One way an athlete can show this respect to her fellow competitors is to engage in practices that promote this interconnectedness, oneness, or interdependence by ensuring that fair play is observed. While competitions are about teams or individuals opposing each other in order to win, the opposition is important as it brings out the best from each competitor. What connects competitors as human beings is more fundamental and stronger than what separates them as opponents in a particular competition. In this case, to use banned drugs or methods in order to win is to emphasise and encourage differences which are contingent because human beings are fundamentally interconnected or interdependent.

Another group of positive values which are central to the Umunthu way of life, and which we think can positively contribute to the prevention of doping, include care, respect, and responsibility. When one recognises the importance of interdependence or interconnectedness, she is more than willing to care for, respect, and exercise responsibility towards the welfare of others. Through the caring attitude, one treats the well-being of others with whom he or she shares the social space with respect. To be responsible is to be virtuous or do something honourable. Within the Umunthu framework, anyone who does not care about others but opts to live for himself or herself is not a Munthu (person) for he or she is violating the rules of living together as one people. To say one is not a Munthu is not to suggest that one is not a human being. Rather, it simply means this individual is not humane enough to transcend physical existence to become a moral person. Responsibility is the basis of togetherness of humanity. In sports, if an athlete or a player recognises this requirement of Umunthu, namely, that human beings are one, then he or she is receptive to the ideas of care and respect others. In the sporting world, that care or respect ultimately consists in avoiding illegal or unethical means for winning such as performance-enhancing substances and methods.

One way of showing respect, care, and responsibility towards fellow athletes is to engage in practices that ensure fair play for all individual athletes or teams participating in a given competition. Fair play includes athletes adhering to the established laws of the game, such as the anti-doping laws whose primary aim is to level the playing field for all players as well as safeguard the spirit of sports. The use of performance-enhancing drugs and methods shows selfishness and does not promote equality of all players or the spirit of sports. What makes sports interesting is the unpredictability of results. Those who use performance-enhancing substances and methods emphasise on individuality and gamesmanship, which take away this very soul of sports. With individuality and gamesmanship, athletes cannot exercise responsibility towards one another. An athlete who possesses Umunthu attitude is capable of showing compassion, reciprocity, mutuality, and caring for her fellow athletes. Abisha Mugari (2021, p. 21) has argued that although cheating in sport is a common practice which has continued to rob sporting competitions of their attraction, this practice defies the expectations of the authentic person from an African perspective. Umunthu qualities would prevent one from practising doping.

Kindness and generosity are also critical values within the Umunthu philosophy. Within Umunthu, acts of kindness and generosity are regarded as the foundation upon which rests the notion of sharing, which is itself a critical idea in the life of community. To be a true Munthu is to be generous with one's resources, both material and immaterial. As a virtue, generosity is a sign of selflessness which enables people to stand together in want or plenty. In their early life, and through various legendary stories and proverbs, children are taught the importance of sharing as a very important Umunthu or communitarian value. Sharing is one way of expressing oneness, bondedness, and selflessness. Since sharing will naturally occur as an important virtue of community living, it actually becomes the organising logic that holds communities together.

From the three clusters of Umunthu values, emphasis has been laid on values such as kindness, generosity, respect, caring, and responsibility towards each other. These values which are pervasive within communal settings help individuals become more humane. This will likely lead individuals in the community, in our case athletes, to develop strong bonds with one another. Umunthu therefore transcends the narrow confines of the nuclear family where love and commitment are extended only to the kinship network. Such an attitude or behaviour is critical for the prevention of doping in sports. Beyond winning, athletes should primarily be concerned about the welfare of others and how they can contribute to good life of all members in the community since all actions have an impact on other members of the society. The elements of Umunthu value system or philosophy moderate the behaviour of athletes in any sporting competition as responsibility becomes the basis of togetherness of humanity.

2.8 Conclusion

Thus far, we have been trying to demonstrate the critical role that Umunthu philosophy or value system can play in various anti-doping initiatives. Specifically, Umunthu philosophy is capable of becoming a framework underlying the anti-doping initiatives. In our demonstration, we have explained how WADA fulfils its obligations as the main anti-doping authority. To appreciate the problem of doping, we have explored the nature of sports through human nature. Specifically, doping behaviour can be traced to the selfish human nature as aptly interrogated in Thomas Hobbes' philosophy. Again, to appreciate the significance of various anti-doping drives, we laboured to show why doping in sports is unethical. We touched on WADA's priority areas in its anti-doping work. This was meant to show some limitations and why the Umunthu framework we are suggesting here should be seriously considered. We endeavoured to provide a brief discussion of what the Umunthu philosophy is about before focusing on some selected elements to demonstrate their viability as the basis of anti-doping initiatives which in our view can make a significant contribution to the prevention of doping in sports in Africa and beyond. In this chapter we emphasised the qualities of Umunthu as a perspective complementing the anti-doping efforts by WADA.

References

Aicinena, S. (2010). Sport as war or a means to peace? Thomas Hobbes' laws of nature. *International Journal of Business and Social Science, 1*(1), 15–25.

Archer, A. (2016). On sporting integrity. *Sport, Ethics and Philosophy, 10*(2), 117–131. https// doi.org/10.1080/17511321.2016.1140223

Baron, D. A, Martin, D. M., and Magd, S. A. (2007). Doping in sports and its spread to at-risk populations: an international review. *World Psychiatry*, 6(2), 118–123.

Bloodworth, A. (2018). A philosophical response to the critics of anti-doping. Retrieved February 2, 2023 from https://idrottsforum.org/bloand_murray180618/

Bloodworth, A. J., and McNamee, M. (2017). Sport, society, and anti-doping policy: An ethical overview. In O. Rabin and Y. Pitsiladis (Eds.), *Medicine and Sport Science: Volume 62. Acute Topics in Anti-Doping*. Basel: Karger Publishers (pp. 177–185). https://doi.org/10.1159/000460748

Boyacıoğlu, F., and Oğuz, A.G. (2016). The role of sports in international relations. *Acta Universitatis Danubius. Relationes Internationales, 9*(1), 99–108.

Caplan, A. L., and Parent, B. (Eds.) (2017). *Ethics of Sport: Essential Readings*. New York: Oxford University Press.

Chigangaidze, R. K. and Chinyenze, P. (2022). What it means to say, 'a person is a person through other persons': Ubuntu through humanistic-existential lenses of transactional analysis. *Journal of Religion & Spirituality in Social Work: Social Thought, 41*(3), 280–295. https://doi.org/10.1080/15426432.2022.2039341

Chigangaidze, R. K., Matanga, A. A., and Katsuro, T. R. (2022). Ubuntu philosophy as a humanistic–existential framework for the fight against the COVID-19 pandemic. *Journal of Humanistic Psychology, 62*(3), 319–333. https://doi.org/10.1177/00221678211044554

Dvorak, J., Saugy, M., and Pitsiladis, Y. P. (2014). Challenges and threats to implementing the fight against doping in sport. *British Journal of Sports Medicine, 48*, 807–809. https://doi.org/10.1136/bjsports-2014-093589

Fouché, R. (2012). Aren't athletes cyborgs? Technology, bodies, and sporting competitions. *Women's Studies Quarterly, 40* (1/2), 281–293.

Gamage, K. A. A., Dehideniya, D. M. S. C. P. K., and Ekanayake, S. Y. (2021). The role of personal values in learning approaches and student achievements. *Behavioural Sciences, 11*, 1–23. https://doi.org/10.3390/bs11070102

Gatterer, K., Gumpenberger, M., Overbye, M., Streicher, B., Schobersberger, W., and Blank, C. (2020). An evaluation of prevention initiatives by 53 national anti-doping organisations: achievements and limitations. *Journal of Sports and Health Science, 9*, 228–239.

Ibrahim, L. Y. (2016). Integrity issues in competitive sports. *Journal of Sports and Physical Education (IOSR-JSPE), 3*(5), 67–72.

Isidori, E., and Benetton, M. (2015). Sport as education: between dignity and human rights. *Procedia – Social and Behavioral Sciences, 197*, 686–693.

Merriam, C. E. (1906). Hobbes's doctrine of the state of nature. *Proceedings of the American Political Science Association, 3*, 151–157.

Mugari, A. (2021). Unbundling the nexus of sport cheating: leveraging on the philosophy of Hunhuism/Ubuntuism. *Global Journal of Arts Humanity and Social Sciences, 1*(1), 21–27.

Murove, F. M. (2012). Ubuntu. *Diogenes, 59*(3/4), 36–47. https://doi.org/10.1177/0392192113493737

Murray, T. H. (2017). A moral foundation for anti-doping: how far have we progressed? Where are the limits? *Medicine and Sport Science, 62*, 186–193. https://doi.org/10.1159/000460749

Palmi, I., Berretta, P., Tini, A., Ricci, G., and Marinelli, S. (2019). The unethicality of doping in sports. *La Clinica Terapeutica, 170*(2), e100–e101. https://doi.org/10.7417/CT.2019.2117

Peskov, A. (2019). Problems of the fight against doping in professional sports: on the example of Russian and world experience. In K. Margaritis (Ed.), *Law, Ethics, and Integrity in the Sports Industry*. Pennsylvania: IGI Global (pp. 202–240)..

Pisk, J. (2011). Sport: the treasure of temperance. *Physical Culture and Sport. Studies and Research, 51*(1), 53–61. https://doi.org/10.2478/v10141-011-0005-9

Schneider, A. J., and Friedmann, T. (2006). The problem of doping in sports. In J. C. Hall, J. C. Dunlap, T. Friedmann, and V. van Heyningen (Eds.), *Advances in Genetics: Volume 51. Gene Doping in Sports: The Science and Ethics of Genetically Modified Athletes*. Cambridge, MA: Academic Press (pp. 1–9). https://doi.org/10.1016/S0065-2660(06)51001-6

Sebri, V., Savioni, L., Triberti, S., Mazzocco, K., and Pravettoni, G. (2019). How to train your health: sports as a resource to improve cognitive abilities in cancer patients. *Frontiers in Psychology, 10*, 1–10. https://doi.org/10.3389/fpsyg.2019.02096

Simon, R. L. (2016). *The Ethics of Sport: What Everyone Needs to Know*. New York: Oxford University Press.

Stewart, C. C. (2014). Sportsmanship, gamesmanship, and the implications for coach education. *Strategies, 27*(5), 3–7. https://doi.org/10.1080/08924562.2014.938878

Vorstenbosch, J. (2010). Doping and cheating. *Journal of the Philosophy of Sport, 37*(2), 166–181. https://doi.org/10.1080/00948705.2010.9714774

WADA. (2017). WADA Ethics Panel: guiding values in sport and anti-doping. Retrieved January 20, 2023 from www.wada-ama.org/sites/default/files/resources/files/wada_ethicspanel_setofnorms_oct2017_en.pdf

Wright, J., and Jayawickrama, J. (2021). "We need other human beings in order to be human": examining the indigenous philosophy of Umunthu and strengthening mental health interventions. *Culture, Medicine, and Psychiatry, 45*, 613–628. https://doi.org/10.1007/s11013-020-09692-4

Chapter 3

The African Athlete and Contemporary Francophone Fiction

Doping in Jean-Marc Rigaux's *Kipjiru 42… 195*

Beaton Galafa

3.1 Introduction

The existence and use of alleged performance-enhancing substances have remained well known among sports workers for decades in modern history and are a global menace in the sporting world (Bale, 2009; Soita, 2017). With the central role occupied by sports in political and economic spaces, any scandals characterising its activities receive critical attention. The significance of sports in elevating the status of states has often led to systemic doping worldwide. From the infamous East German doping scheme (the 1960s–1980s) to the four-year ban on Russian athletes by the World Anti-Doping Agency (WADA) and Global Sports in 2021, we get to understand performance enhancement as playing an almost omnipresent role in sports (He, 2022; Dimeo et al., 2011). Notably, the omnipresence of doping has led to its fictionalisation.

Due to the inspiration that fiction draws from human experiences, any infamous sporting scandals such as doping would be the birth of scintillating works of sports fiction, giving an ordinary reader a window into the nitty-gritty of such malpractices. In general, literary responses to sports have seen the rise of sports fiction in entirely different periods, albeit slowly (Sheehan, 2020). Nevertheless, there has already been a literary turn in sports studies, with scholars considering literary, poetic, and dramatic modes of recording their research while exploring the contents of extant literature to interpret the world of sports and their representations (Bale, 2009, p. 190). Some outstanding examples spread across time include Knud Lundberg's *The Olympic Hope* (1958), Peter May's *The Runner* (2003), and S.B. Divya's *Machinehood* (2021).

While we would expect at least a near-similar response in African fiction, a quick search hits a blank wall. However, a little more adventure and we stumble on Jean-Marc Rigaux's *Kipjiru 42… 195*. The novel is an enquiry by an unnamed protagonist and narrator into the death of a Ugandan athlete, John Kipjiru, in the town of Eldoret in Kenya. This chapter, therefore, explores how *Kipjiru 42… 195* develops the narrative of doping in Africa as the protagonist

DOI: 10.4324/9781003370796-4

discovers how deeply entrenched the practice is in marathon racing in East Africa. A significant part of the story occurs in Kenya and Uganda, although dramatic scenes are spread across Europe and East Africa. In the novel, John Kipjiru, a famous world champion runner originally from Uganda, is assassinated at his apartment in Eldoret, Kenya. A gruesome scene: Kipjiru is circumcised post-murder and has his feet cut off. His assassination becomes the centre of an investigation by a world athletics body, the Union Mondiale Athlétique (UMA), with the organisation's primary concern being establishing and destroying any links between the assassination and doping. Voiturier (2022, para. 2) argues that the novel:

> nous entraîne à pénétrer dans les coulisses de ces clans plus ou moins occultes qui régissent le sport de haut niveau et, notamment, ceux qui sont censés lutter contre le dopage ainsi que ceux qui trament des actions plus ou moins licites au niveau international afin de manipuler des athlètes en vue d'arrangements clandestins.
>
> (takes us behind the scenes of the more or less occult clans that govern the high-level sport, particularly those who are supposed to fight against doping and those who plot more or less legal actions at the international level to manipulate athletes for clandestine arrangements.)

In Rigaux's demonstration of the gravity of doping, the novel further introduces us to genetic research of pharmaceutical laboratories to increase human performance to benefit shareholders in the sport.

As a Belgian author, his novel becomes particularly interesting to the African reader because it is primarily set in Africa, with a theme that gives us insights into doping in African marathon racing. By reading *Kipjiru 42... 195*, this chapter charts an interpretation of the world of athletics in Africa and its representation of doping. The chapter draws perspectives on the African athlete and doping in marathon racing through the eyes of the protagonist in the novel. A reading of the representation of doping in the novel is aided by three specific objectives, namely: (1) to set *Kipjiru 42... 195* as a window into our understanding of African doping in Francophone fiction, (2) to locate direct and indirect doping references in the novel, and (3) to establish the connection between fiction and reality in doping in the context of athletics as presented in the novel.

The chapter treats *Kipjiru 42... 195* as a work of Francophone African fiction, mainly due to the rarity of African literary fiction themed around doping. Thus, the choice of *Kipjiru 42... 195*, apart from its theme and experience, which are relevant to the African context, is a consequence of the paucity of African literary works that engage doping in its World Anti-Doping Agency (WADA) sense. Further, the chapter compensates for this lack by exploiting memory as deployed in the novel to understand doping in athletics and its African context. The chapter's exploration of the novel also maintains relevance due to literature's ability to traverse borders regardless of the author's identity. This permits the chapter to have an open and in-depth engagement with Jean-Marc Rigaux's representation of doping in the African context. The critical reading of *Kipjiru 42... 195* is aided by available scholarly texts on doping in Francophone African literature.

3.2 Doping in Francophone Fiction

Since the invention of sports, the desire to win has always driven sporting personalities to resort to doping. *Mon père, sa mère*, a novel by Thierry Bellefroid, sarcastically introduces us to an important temporal concept relating to doping: "The Greeks have nothing left to prove, they invented the Olympic Games and therefore doping..." (Bellefroid, 2006, p. 11). Pinpointing the inseparable nature of the two highlights the strong nexus between athletics and doping that has become an archetype of sports fiction in Francophone writing. It is unsurprising, therefore, to encounter the existence of numerous novels on sports in which doping takes centre stage in Francophone literature.

Florent Dabadie's *À revers*, for example, takes readers into a merciless world of top-level sport. Between parental ambition, the sacrifice of youth, and the slippage into doping, this novel explores a thrilling world as it reveals the implacable workings of one of the greatest scourges of contemporary sport (Dabadie, 2020). The doping motif in Francophone fiction resurfaces in *Trop fort tony!* by Eric Simard. In the novel, on the eve of the Rio Olympics and the European Football Cup in 2016, a man offers the protagonist Tony a doping product that should enable him to score incredible goals. He falls for the offer, and the goals he scores render him a star (Simard, 2016). However, the plot twists to the hazards of doping when the protagonist's health becomes compromised, compelling Tony to quit doping.

Doping is also recurring in *Les Olympiades truquées* by Joëlle Wintrebert and Jean-Noël Blanc's *Le Tour de France n'aura pas lieu*. The former centres on a protagonist who is an exceptional swimmer. A rising star and prospective champion of approaching Olympic games, a doping incident turns her violent and leads to experiences that see her wanting to regain control of her mind and body (Wintrebert, 2001). Similarly, *Le Tour de France n'aura pas lieu*'s plot is built around the seizure of prohibited products in the car of two riders and the doping-related death of one of the cyclists on the eve of the Tour de France (Blanc, 2000). All this convinces the main character Tavernier of a doping culture in cycling, which leads into the novel's series of experiences as he pursues the truth.

This existence of a comparatively vast repertoire of fiction that dwells on doping experiences may be a direct result of open and direct conversations on doping in the Western world. It is also a reflection of how much western writing has evolved in its literary genres, producing fascinating works in sports fiction (Sheehan, 2020). Rigaux's *Kipjiru 42... 195*, with its doping theme, exists within this context. However, what differentiates the novel from the sampled Francophone works is that although Rigaux sets it in various places across Europe and Africa, his primary target appears to be doping in African athletics. This realisation is derived from the fact that much of the scintillating action either takes places in Africa or involves greater participation of African characters, in addition to the fact that the whole novel centres on Kipjiru, a Ugandan athlete assassinated in Kenya.

3.3 The African Athlete and Doping

Since the chapter's focus rests on the representation of the African athlete and doping in Francophone African fiction, understanding such a work would require an exploration of the real-life African doping terrain. It is thus imperative that before navigating any possible literary output as a product of the vice, we chronicle some recorded activity pertaining to what Bale (2009, p. 191) terms "the application of scientific methods to the deviant athletic body". Such chronicling helps in locating African narratives of doping within their fictional representation.

Within African literature, the emphasis on *Juju* means doping has often failed to appear as the primary focus in narratives that dwell on achievement performance in sports. In what is called spiritual doping, sporting characters on the continent often highlight the superimposition of the spiritual and material worlds as the principal motivation for *Juju* (Kovač, 2018). Despite this being the case, sporting activities such as athletics, a successful discipline in African participation in the racing space, remain permeated by realities of doping in the WADA's sense.

In East Africa, a popular terrain in the world of athletics, doping revelations have repeatedly appeared on the international scene. For example, a report from Germany's Zweites Deutsches Fernsehen in 2019 alleged that top athletes in Kenya regularly used the endurance-boosting substance Erythropoïétines (EPO) in training (DW, 2019). Moreover, as of August 2021, Kenya was pegged at the summit of a table of athletes banned for doping violations – only second to Russia (*The Economist*, 2021). In 2011, an Ethiopian runner Ezkyas Sisay was suspended for two years after testing positive to EPO at the New York City marathon (Olivier, 2015). As is the case with Kenya, the suspensions in Ethiopia have also been recurring, especially in the past decade.

While East Africa features greatly in doping narratives on the continent owing to its place in long-distance marathon, performance enhancement remains a recurring reality throughout the continent. In South Africa, for example, rugby and cycling have come out as sporting activities deeply rooted in doping, with the Springboks 1995 World Cup victory raising doping suspicions years later (Soumaré, 2019). Similarly, other big sporting countries on the continent have had their fair share of doping, with Nigerian sprinters also featuring highly, at some point resulting in a stripping of medals won at the African Games (Diawara, 2016). These few highlighted cases reflect what has become a major problem among sporting personalities on the continent. However, long-distance running occupies a special place in the African doping discourse because it is one of the very few areas in which African athletes enjoy dominance.

3.4 Any Literary Response?

Ideally, an African author would be better placed to offer insights into the African creative perception of doping in sports on the continent. However, the recurrence of doping scandals on the continent has not triggered any promptly visible response in its literary writing. The continent's oeuvre on the theme, if any, has tended to tilt towards the ethno-spiritual narratives of *Juju* in lieu of the known established concept of doping. Nonetheless, this does not point to a total lack of sports fiction on the continent, with the presence of novels such as *Don't Die on Wednesday* by Michael Afenfia (Murua, 2019). Narrowing the gaze towards Francophone African writing is painstakingly fruitless, at least in the meantime. As such, with doping largely remaining an underexplored (if not unexplored) theme, a quest for Francophone fiction that features doping requires a relatively wider cast of the net.

3.5 A Rare Francophone Fiction Window

Jean-Marc Rigaux's *Kipjiru 42...195* offers a rare literary window into the Francophone novel's representation and interpretation of the African athlete in marathon running on multiple levels. The novel's unnamed protagonist, a former lawyer and specialist in the Rwandan genocide, is sent to the field to secretly investigate for the Union Mondiale Athletique (UMA) – a sports federation headquartered in Monaco (Rigaux, 2020). He is sent because of his African experience in the International Criminal Tribunal for Rwanda, a fact we are repeatedly reminded of through his flashbacks as he draws parallels with the unpleasant experiences he encounters on his quest for answers. In one dramatic scene after the other, we traverse cities and countries: Monaco, Nairobi, Eldoret, Liège, Goslar, London, Brussels, Uganda (with its cities, towns, and villages), and Kenya (again – after the Nairobi stint earlier).

In a series of main escapades, the protagonist has a connection from the UMA, an old-time friend he shares the racing passion with called Léon, who guides him. However, the protagonist-narrator briefly loses contact in Goslar where he is implicated in the murder of Kaltbrück, the late Kipjiru's manager whom he was investigating (Rigaux, 2020). On their reconnection after another brief escapade in London (where he was investigating big pharma companies and their laboratories in connection with Kipjiru's assassination), he learns that the mission is over. Léon is expendable (Rigaux, 2020, p. 203).

The UMA does not have anything to do with the protagonist, provided that he keeps himself away from the organisation. Following Léon's death, the protagonist is forced to flee to Uganda. Here, a part of him believes he will find a final piece to the Kipjiru puzzle. He also wishes to marry Eurydice – a Kenyan female runner who had earlier served as his primary contact in Eldoret where he previously broke into Kipjiru's apartment.

Through his globetrotting encounters which culminate in the protagonist finally settling in Kenya in the novel's resolution, Rigaux introduces us to a foreigner's gaze on the African athletic landscape. Further and more important is the protagonist's exceptional connoisseur character of African life that he ends up being circumcised and accepted into the Kalenjin tribe (Rigaux, 2020, p. 324). The immersion that happens in the last chapter as well as the character's continuous display of knowledge of the African people aids in constructing powerful narratives around doping, keeping the plot lively to the reader throughout. Rigaux thus builds a character that evades scrutiny when the protagonist-narrator uncovers grand schemes of doping that parallel real-life doping scandals of modern history in Africa. Thus, *Kipjiru 42… 195* presents itself as a very rare window of Francophone fiction into the African doping story.

3.6 Doping in *Kipjiru 42… 195*

In *Kipjiru 42… 195*, Rigaux directly confronts doping in East African marathon racing through a particular storyline that starts with murder. He is certain that for those in the marathon industry, doping is a well-known widespread activity. While sustaining this position in the entire plot, Rigaux also superimposes his thought through the exchanges his protagonist-narrator has with various characters, such as a retired runner, Chepgat, in Eldoret and Kaltbrück in Goslar. Chepgat reveals the use of performance-enhancing pills/drugs behind the curtain, calling them "les medicines des Blancs" (Rigaux, 2020, p. 98). He admits having engaged in doping himself. However, he is quick to state that the drugs are not taken by every athlete because they are very expensive and are only offered to promising athletes as a reward. This comes out clear in a conversation on doping between Chepgat and the protagonist when the latter queries on what happens behind the curtain:

- Je ne sais pas moi-même. Il y a des choses, Les médecines des Blancs.
- Les « médecines »?
- Oui, je n'avais pas grand-chose à faire. Kaltbrück me demandait de préparer les pilules et les piqures.
- Les pilules et les piqures? (Rigaux, 2020, p. 98)

(- I don't know myself. There are things, White People's Medicines.
- The "medicines"?

- Yes, I didn't have much to do. Kaltbrück asked me to prepare pills and injections.
- Pills and injections?)

On the last question, Chepgat gives us more insights into the depth of the doping. Rigaux, through Chepgat, presents the image of doping as a highly systematic exercise that is perpetrated even by managers of the athletes. The former athlete believes the UMA in this context was even paying a blind eye to doping:

> J'en ai pris moi-même dès que j'ai un manager. La fédération, à l'époque, ne s'occupait pas de ça. Quand un talent émergeait, il se mariait à un manager.
>
> (Rigaux, 2020, p. 98)

> (I took them myself as soon as I had a manager. The federation, at that time, didn't deal with that. When a talent emerged, he got himself a manager.)

When asked on whether Kipjiru – the assassinated champion – engaged in doping, Chepgat denied any such knowledge. However, he highlighted that Kipjiru was a champion, and therefore that could have indicated doping though such an assertion proved nothing: "Je ne sais pas. Il a été champion olympique. C'est une indication. Pas une preuve" (I don't know. He was an Olympic champion. That's an indication. Not proof.) (Rigaux, 2020, p. 99). Later, as the protagonist (working undercover as a journalist) interviews Kaltbrück, the latter calls doping "passeport à médailles" (the passport to medals) (Rigaux, 2020, p. 100). The revelations in these two contexts, and the recurring references to doping scandals around the world, reinforce in the reader the image of doping as a well-sanctioned practice in the world of sports.

Rigaux also creates the impression of a doping empire that fights back when confronted. In the novel, the protagonist's leads leave a trail of bodies. Kipjiru's assassination at the outset is just the beginning of a string of violence and death that mark the investigation. First, the protagonist survives an assassination attempt at the Nairobi Museum. But the real post-Kipjiru assassinations start in Goslar, when the protagonist returns to Kaltbrück's house for a clandestine room search. As he traverses rooms, he encounters a dead Kaltbrück in the kitchen – shot on the forehead (Rigaux, 2020, p. 160). We learn later through his exchanges with Léon that this murder was the work of Fausto – a professional assassin who had followed the protagonist throughout his endeavours, contracted by UMA. Kaltbrück is murdered for his knowledge of the doping cartel, and his plans to fight them. We know this through Kaltbrück himself who believes that it was the UMA that murdered Kipjiru and promises to bring the organisation down (Rigaux, 2020, p. 145). The protagonist finds Kaltbrück's evidence against the UMA in a red book he [Kaltbrück] kept hidden in a room with an iron door in which under the first sub-chapter Kaltbrück documents revelations and evidence of managers, officials, and everyone involved in doping with the drugs they used/whose use they facilitated – managers, agents, doctors, sporting clubs, pharmaceutical companies, laboratories (Rigaux, 2020, p. 158). In the same book, we learn that:

> La deuxième sous-chemise traitait la couverture de ces trafics par certains organes d'institutions. En était-on informe au plus haut niveau ? Ce n'était pas sûr. On ne pouvait nier qu'au moins des membres éminents de l'UMA, de fédérations, d'agences anti-dopage était au courant de beaucoup d'éléments de la première sous-chemise.
>
> (Rigaux, 2020, p. 158)

> (The second sub-chapter dealt with the cover-up of such trafficking by certain institutional bodies. Were they informed at the highest level? It was not certain. It could not be denied that at least senior members of the UMA, federations, anti-doping agencies were aware of many elements of the first sub-chapter.)

After the murder of Kaltbrück, Léon is the second victim. In their meeting in Brussels, the protagonist learns all the secrets from Léon, who informs him that he is sharing all because he is already dead – expendable. He knows that Fausto will murder him, and calling the police is useless as the organisation will simply send another Fausto:

> Bien sûr. Il y aura toujours un autre Fausto pour achever son travail. Je suis déjà mort. C'est pour ça que je voudrais courir une dernière fois avec toi demain.
>
> (Rigaux, 2020, p. 203)

> (Of course. There will always be another Fausto to complete its work. I am already dead. That's why I'd like to run with you one last time tomorrow.)

The prophecy is fulfilled as they race together reminiscent of their olden days. Léon is assassinated, in the same way as Kaltbrück by Fausto (p. 215). Ironically, Fausto is himself murdered by three Ugandan security agents who had also been tailing the protagonist. This reveals the complex nature of Kipjiru's case. Having developed doping as the overarching theme, Rigaux successfully completes the picture of a dangerous but lucrative affair. In the words of Kaltbrück, "Le dopage? C'est toute une affaire" (Doping? It's a big deal) (Rigaux, 2020, p. 140). Following the deaths in Brussels, Rigaux takes the reader to Uganda where the protagonist flees to.

Here, he is kidnapped and tortured by security agents attempting to extract information on whether Kipjiru indulged in doping. However, it does not take long before his captors are themselves killed by another group of state security agents linked to his three stalkers (Rigaux, 2020, p. 231). The three stalkers transfer him to the Ministry of Defense headquarters (Rigaux, 2020, p. 231). The involvement of the UMA and the state security agents in the spate of murders that characterise the dramatic action in the novel serves to uncover systemic operations sanctioned by high-level powers. In Liège, Léon had already explained the Ugandan state's interest in discovering the truth behind Kipjiru's murder. Referring to the murder's cause, he said: "Une autre option, c'est le dopage. Si Kipjiru en était convaincu, ce serait un désastre pour l'Ouganda. D'où la nécessité de tirer cela au clair" (Another option is doping. If Kipjiru was convinced [and therefore resorted to doping], it would be a disaster for Uganda. Hence the need to get to the bottom of it) (Rigaux, 2020, p. 117). From deaths and the surrounding circumstances that we encounter in the novel, Rigaux presents the complexities of doping as a regular occurrence with an organised system that is ready to defend its existence at all cost.

Rigaux highlights the existence of a large-scale systemic doping cable. This is very evident from Kaltbrück's chronicles in his secret red book (Rigaux, 2020, p. 158). It also corroborates Léon's argument much earlier that all top runners engage in doping – with the UMA itself being composed of the same top athletes. In their discussion of the protagonist's reports on Kipjiru's assassination, Léon problematises the concept of doping as being endemic even in the UMA:

> Le dopage, c'est aussi une précaution. On ne sait jamais.
> - Qu'est-ce que tu en penses pour Kipjiru?
> - Rien. La question n'est pas si. La question est dans quelles conditions?
> - L'UMA sait que tout le haut niveau est ...?
> - L'UMA est composée d'athlètes de haut niveau.
>
> (Rigaux, 2020, p. 126)

> (Doping is also a precaution. You never know.
> - What do you think about Kipjiru?
> - Nothing. The question is not whether. The question is under what conditions?
> - Does UMA know that all the top level is...?
> - UMA is made up of top athletes.)

But even before that, the very first meeting that Léon arranges between the protagonist and the three anonymous members of the UMA in Brussels is already revealing. Rigaux, through the narrator, creates the impression of this meeting as a mafia meeting: "Je m'étais imaginé, pendant que Léon me faisait son briefing, me retrouver dans une atmosphère de réunion mafieuse [...]" (I had imagined, while Léon was briefing me, that I was in a mafia meeting atmosphere) (Rigaux, 2020, p. 21). By sharing this reflection, Rigaux sets the tone of doping as a dangerous criminal affair from the onset. The first UMA member speaks of the need for the organisation to investigate the cause of Kipjiru's death. On a suggested list of possible causes, doping appears first. This points to doping as an obvious criminal activity in the sport. The organisation highlights the possibility of destroying evidence and distracting the media in the event where undesirable results are obtained. Léon urges his friend to understand the UMA simply as powerful people with means of attaining their objectives (Rigaux, 2020, p. 27).

Throughout the novel, Rigaux demonstrates the unshifting position of the organisation's desire to keep things quiet, where in the end Kipjiru remains a hero – untainted by any possible doping suspicions. In Brussels, Léon confirms with the protagonist that his findings that Kipjiru was murdered are true since the UMA also found the same: "On a fait les comparaisons avec les données que nous possedions. C'est bien Kipjiru a été assassiné" (We made comparisons with the data we had. It is true that Kipjiru was murdered) (Rigaux, 2020, p. 113). The narrator also learns from Léon that his mission is over, and that findings from his investigation will remain a secret, with Kipjiru's heroic figure remaining unscathed (Rigaux, 2020, p. 200). This ending also resonates with outcomes of the protagonist's encounters with the Ugandan state security agents. Once he is in Uganda, the protagonist unexpectedly attains freedom to be a Ugandan national – but he is also allowed freedom to relocate to an East African country of his choice. He is taken to Hotel Serena right in the capital, Kampala, on government bills (Rigaux, 2020, pp. 234–236). Given VIP treatment, the security agents and the government completely leave the protagonist alone to the extent that any later attempts on his life do not attract the government's attention as would normally be the case considering his preceding importance to the authorities (Rigaux, 2020, p. 313). This sudden disinterest from the state emerges upon noticing that the protagonist failed to uncover Kipjiru's murderer or indeed whether the latter engaged in doping as a marathon champion.

Through the doctor sent by Léon to the narrator as he quits the London pharma labs assignment for Goslar, we learn of highly secretive experiments (including genetic experimentation) that would revolutionise the doping industry. In his explanation of the experiments at Genetic Solutions, the doctor tells the narrator that:

> Le dopage génétique est la clé qui peut ouvrir ou fermer la porte de toutes ces vanités. Un État ou une compagnie peut rendre plus ou moins égal un sujet donné, ou fantasme suprême, donner les mêmes gènes à tous.
>
> (Rigaux, 2020, p. 189)

(Genetic doping is the key that can open or close the door to all these vanities. A state or a company can make a given subject more or less equal, or in the highest of fantasies, give the same genes to all.)

A break-in at Genetic Solutions in London by the protagonist, who flees Goslar after the assassination of Kaltbrück, reveals a lot of genetic projects in the lab. The doctor he meets later – a messenger from Léon in Brussels – discloses the intentions of some of the projects, notable among them a doping project (the EPO) that would render the whole anti-doping control efforts inefficient. He explains to the protagonist that with the EPO, "Pour les sportifs, c'est l'idéal. La barrière de votre manufacture de globules rouges est brisée. Le contrôle anti-dopage inefficient. Liberté chérie" (For athletes, this is ideal. The barrier of your red blood cell manufacture is broken. Anti-doping control ineffective. Freedom dear) (Rigaux, 2020, p. 186). This conversation signals how highly systemic the whole doping business is – with mass investment by big pharmaceuticals. While we might not be privy to how close or far from reality the position as advanced in the novel is in the nonfiction world, we at least get a clear idea of the different players in the doping business. It is here, in the exchanges between the doctor and the protagonist, that we learn of the principal role assumed by big pharma companies in taking doping to entirely new levels.

3.7 The Nexus between Fiction and Reality

Kipjiru 42… 195 achieves the connection between fiction and reality through allusion to real doping scandals, existence of real political systems, and reference to historical happenings as well as cultural and traditional events in the East African context. But how much of what Rigaux highlights would we say represents the place of doping in African marathon racing? As argued by Goldbort (1995, p. 88), the unique contribution of fiction to the study of scientific ethics is that, in presenting parallel worlds, it not only reflects reality but judges it. The unfolding events in *Kipjiru 42… 195* place us in a suitable position where we are either reminded of the realities of doping in marathon racing or tempted to imagine the clandestine underpinnings around the activity. Rigaux achieves this by entwining the novel's plot with infamous factual happenings in the sports world.

From the very beginning, the protagonist's guess of the three anonymous UMA members locates them as of Russian and East African origin (Rigaux, 2020, pp. 21–23). In situating these characters in the exposition, Rigaux creates a context for a real link between fiction and nonfiction that develops along with the story throughout. The Russian-African connection is a reminder of the history and contemporaneity of doping in world athletics. Highlighting the politics of sport, Léon alludes to state-sponsored doping in communist regimes (Rigaux, 2020, p. 123), a historical reality of the infamous

East German doping scandals in the history of Olympics (Dimeo et al., 2011). Léon, when asked whether the UMA knows that all athletes at the high level engage in doping, responds by saying the organisation is made of former top athletes (Rigaux, 2020, p. 126). Likewise, Rigaux's use of allusion pays off when he draws the reader's attention to the German journalist Hans-Joachim Seppelt who uncovered widespread doping practices by Kenyan athletes in a 2012 documentary (Kelsall, 2012). This he achieves through the character of Kaltbrück who narrates everything as illustrated in that report/documentary on German television:

> La télé allemande a fait un reportage l'an dernier. Atterrant ! C'était un petit futé ce Hans Joachim Seppelt. Caméra cachée. Se présentant en agent de coureurs européens. On lui a tout expliqué, ou aller, quelles officines, quels produits, comment prendre, quelles techniques pour éviter de se faire prendre. On voyait tout.
>
> (Rigaux, 2020, p. 139)

> (German TV did a report last year. Astonishing! Hans Joachim Seppelt was a smart guy. Hidden camera. Presenting himself as an agent for European runners. He was told everything, where to go, which shops, which products, how to take them, which techniques to avoid being caught. We could see everything).

Kaltibruck further alludes to a doping scandal of Chinese athletes in the 1990s (see Chavez, 2017) as he attempts to clarify that doping did not start with the Kenyans. He urges the narrator to "Notez que les Kenyans n'ont pas été les premiers. Rappelez-vous les chinois dans les annees 1990" (Note that the Kenyans were not the first. Remember the Chinese in the 1990s) (Rigaux, 2020, p. 140). This is a direct engagement with the reader's memory on the existence of doping in the nonfiction world, even at the global level.

Further, in thickening the plot to actively involve unsuspicious players in the doping affair, Rigaux ironically brings us closer to reality. While having the UMA, the feds, agents, and managers all entangled in doping may appear as pure fiction rarely present outside *Kipjiru 42... 195*, a careful attention to the realities of athletics in Africa points to the contrary. In 2016, the International Association of Athletics Federations (IAAF) suspended Kenya's Olympics boss over doping allegations in the heat of the 2016 Rio summer games (Soita, 2017). Similarly, various foreign agents/managers have been charged and others expelled from East Africa over doping allegations in the last decade. On the bigger scale, there have been damning reports putting into question the conduct of officials belonging to state Olympic committees as well as IAAF (Ingle, 2016). All this Rigaux successfully captures in his fictive representation of the African athlete in marathon racing. His ability to engage with memory produces a powerful basis for the novel's existence as a reflection of the deviant African athletic body.

In addition, by setting the novel in real time and space, Rigaux also provides us a whole new dimension from which to second-guess our understanding of reality in marathon racing. The featuring of Iten and its training camp in the novel makes its storyline attain some familiarity with contemporary happenstances in the world of African athletics. In a 2020 interview on what inspired him to write the novel, Rigaux referred to the death of another Kenyan athlete who had a very short-lived glorious experience:

> Ensuite, j'ai voulu en savoir le plus possible, non seulement sur le champion olympique de Londres mais aussi sur son prédécesseur Kenyan qui a eu une courte gloire puisqu'il a été assassiné dans la région d'Eldoret, au Kenya.
>
> (Renette, 2020, p. 10)

> (Then I wanted to know as much as possible, not only about the London Olympic champion but also about his Kenyan predecessor who had a short-lived glory as he was murdered in the Eldoret region, in Kenya.)

Kipjiru 42… 195 predates murders of two Kenyan female athletics bronze medallists from the town, Damaris Muthee Mutua in 2022 and Agnes Tirop in 2021 (BBC, 2022). While these murders are not connected to doping as is Kipjiru's in the novel, the critical insights on doping which Rigaux offers cannot allow us to entirely disregard any such possibilities in the nonfiction world. This is because of the striking resemblance in experiences between the characters in the novel and the real athletes. For example, Kipjiru himself belonged to the Iten Training Camp (Rigaux, 2020, p. 94), which is located in the Kenyan athletic town of Iten – a town which is also home to Mutua and Tirop. Thus, in the novel, Rigaux leads the African reader to a mystery adventure on deaths in marathon racing in both fiction and reality.

Farther from sports, Rigaux engages us deeper into his fiction by drawing parallels between doping and events in the Rwandan genocide. Through the protagonist's flashbacks, there is a recurring reference to the brutal massacres every time he encounters a discomforting violent experience. Rigaux prompts our memory by subtly stressing on doping's lethality as regards immortality of performance and invincibility. He says, for example, that "Les tueurs ne buvaient que le soir. Pas pendant l'action. Ils n'en avaient pas besoin. Ils étaient dopés. Dopés à l'invincibilité, à l'immortalité" (The killers only drank at night. Not during the action. They didn't need to. They were doped. Doped to invincibility, to immortality) (Rigaux, 2020, p. 128). Likewise, parallels are also drawn on the consequences of doping. For the genocidaires, this is experienced through the suffering in Congolese refugee camps of Nyiragongo before some are brought to prisons in Kigali (Rigaux, 2020, p. 128). For the doping athlete, the returns are equally devastating:

> Il allait falloir payer. Le prix serait élevé. Très élevé. [...] Pour l'athlète, il se compte en ménisques broyés, en tendons de chanvre usé, en cancers inconnus, en noires dépressions, en enterrements précoces.
>
> (Rigaux, 2020, p. 128)
>
> (There would be a price to pay. The price would be high. Very high. [...] For the athlete, it would be counted in crushed menisci, in sinews of worn hemp, in unknown cancers, in dark depressions, in early burials.)

The link between fiction and nonfiction in the novel builds space for a mirror of self-reflection in African marathon racing and the recurring doping tendencies. Rigaux offers the African an opportunity to navigate doping narratives with a broader view through experiences generated in the reading of *Kipjiru 42... 195*. In the novel, the African reader has a chance to engage critically with the possibilities of a big cable of deviant personalities that form a powerful doping syndicate bent on producing robotic marathon runners. Such engagement emanates from Rigaux's ability to jog the reader's memory about doping in contemporary African and world history.

3.8 Conclusion

In cognisance of the paucity of Francophone African fiction themed on doping in sports, this chapter finds Jean-Marc Rigaux's *Kipjiru 42... 195* a perfect fit for such fictions. The chapter argues that, through a foreigner's gaze, the novel succeeds in offering the reader significant insights into the world of doping in African marathon racing. This is attained through Rigaux's engagement with the reader's memory by entwining his fiction with reality in the history and contemporaneity of doping. The story's setting gives Rigaux a rare chance to display his knowledge of the African people while at the same time offering the reader an opportunity to stare into a mirror for self-reflection. Thus, the novel permits this introspection despite the dearth of relevant African fiction that would allow for the same. Therefore, the novel remains a dependable and realistic representation and interpretation of the nexus between doping and the athletic African body in marathon racing.

References

Bale, J. (2009). Deviance, doping and Denmark in Knud Lundberg's The Olympic Hope. *Sport in History, 29*(2), 190–211. doi: https://doi.org/10.1080/17460260902872628.

BBC. (2022). *Damaris Muthee Mutua: Kenya police launch manhunt after athlete killed*. Retrieved from www.bbc.com/news/world-africa-61160434

Bellefroid, T. (2006). *Mon père, sa mère*. Bruxelles: Racine.

Blanc, J. -N. (2000). *Le tour de France n'aura pas lieu*. Paris: Seuil.

Chavez, C. (2017, October 24). *Report: 'More Than 10,000' Athletes Doped in 80s and 90s, Former Chinese Doctor Claims. Sports Illustrated*. Retrieved from www.si.com/olympics/2017/10/24/chinese-doping-scandal-1980s-1990s-ard-broadcast

Dabadie, F. (2020). *À revers*. Paris: JC Lattès.

Diawara, M. (2016, January 22). Dopage – Nigeria: retrait de sept médailles gagnées aux Jeux africains. *Le Point*. Retrieved from www.lepoint.fr/sport/dopage-nigeria-retrait-de-sept-medailles-gagnees-aux-jeux-africains-22-01-2016-2011928_26.php

Dimeo, P., Hunt, T. M., & Horbury, R. (2011). The individual and the state: a social historical analysis of the East German 'doping system'. *Sport in History, 31*(2), 218–237. doi: https://doi.org/10.1080/17460263.2011.590026.

DW. (2019, September 23). Doping widespread in Kenya ahead of World Athletics Championships — report. *DW*. Retrieved from https://p.dw.com/p/3Q54J.

Goldbort, R. C. (1995). "How dare you sport thus with life?": Frankensteinian fictions as case studies in scientific ethics. *The Journal of Medical Humanities, 16*(2), 79–91.

He, E. (2022, February 5). What does ROC stand for? And why did Russia get banned from Olympics? *NBC Olympics*. Retrieved from www.nbcolympics.com/news/what-does-roc-stand-and-why-did-russia-get-banned-olympics

Ingle, S. (2016, January 7). IAAF in crisis: a complex trail of corruption that led to the very top. *The Guardian*. Retrieved from www.theguardian.com/sport/2016/jan/07/russia-doping-scandal-corruption-blackmail-athletics-iaaf

Kelsall, C. (2012, October 24). Hajo Seppelt — Kenyan doping exposed. *Athletics Illustrated*. Retrieved from https://athleticsillustrated.com/hajo-seppelt-kenyan-doping-exposed/

Kovač, U. (2018, June 27). Du « juju » dans le foot? Triche et dopage à l'africaine. *The Conversation*. Retrieved from https://theconversation.com/du-juju-dans-le-foot-triche-et-dopage-a-lafricaine-97397

Murua, J. (2019, November 1). Five books that centre on sport written by Africans. *James Murua's Literature Blog*. Retrieved from www.jamesmurua.com/five-books-that-centre-sport-written-by-african-writers/

Olivier, M. (2015, August 11). 10 affaires de dopage qui ont secoué le sport africain. *Jeune Afrique*. Retrieved from www.jeuneafrique.com/255987/societe/sport-tricherie-dix-grandes-affaires-de-dopage-africaines/

Renette, A. (2020, September 04). Kipjiru 42… 195, *Le nouvel ouvrage de Jean-Marc Rigaux. Barreau de Liège – Huy*. Retrieved from https://open.barreaudeliege-huy.be/fr/2020/09/04/kipjiru-42195-le-nouvel-ouvrage-de-jean-marc-rigaux

Rigaux, J. -M. (2020). *Kipjiru 42… 195*. Bruxelles: Murmure des soirs.

Sheehan, D. (2020, August 12). Here are the greatest novels ever written about every sport. *Literary Hub*. Retrieved from https://lithub.com/here-are-the-greatest-novels-ever-written-about-every-sport/

Simard, E. (2016). *Trop fort Tony*! Lausanne: Oskar.

Soita, S. S. (2017). *Sports and Drugs: A Critical Analysis of the Legal Framework on Doping in Kenya*. Strathmore University, Strathmore Law School. Retrieved from https://su-plus.strathmore.edu/handle/11071/5289

Soumaré, M. (2019). *Rugby: en Afrique du Sud, une Coupe du monde dans l'ombre de celle de 1995*. Retrieved from www.jeuneafrique.com/832481/societe/rugby-en-afrique-du-sud-une-coupe-du-monde-dans-lombre-de-celle-de-1995/

The Economist (2021). *Sport is still rife with doping*. Retrieved from www.economist.com/science-and-technology/2021/07/14/sport-is-still-rife-with-doping

Voiturier, M. (2022, March 09). Kipjiru 42… 195: fiction policière, réalité dusport de haut niveau, traficotages politique. Association Européenne d'Études Francophones. Retrieved from https://etudesfrancophones.wordpress.com/2022/03/09/kipjiru-42-195-fiction-policiere-realite-du-sport-de-haut-niveau-traficotages-politique/

Wintrebert, J. (2001). *Les olympiades truquées*. Paris: J'ai Lu.

Chapter 4

Ubuntu/Hunhu Ethics as an Anti-Doping Strategy in Sport

Beullah Matinhira and Tawanda Mbewe

4.1 Introduction

Doping is a complex international issue that the world is grappling with today. Performance-enhancing substances inflict immeasurable harm on athletes' health and societal well-being around the globe. It is against this background that doping raises more ethical concerns and has long-lasting negative consequences for the athlete and society. As such, this chapter aims at harnessing Ubuntu/Hunhu ethics to complement efforts to curb the scourge. The conceptualisation of the African ethics of Ubuntu as a worldview that holds dearly the deepest shared values and beliefs of the community over those of an individual may lead to the development of effective anti-doping strategies. Nolte (2014, p.22) strongly notes that the main focus in formulating an anti-doping strategy has been merely testing athletes, which was made possible by developing test mechanisms to deter doping behaviour in athletes. My point of departure in this chapter proceeds from the cognisance that values are socially constructed and apply socially produced systems of motivation for developing anti-doping strategies because sports systems develop within a social context and are socially constructed (Krüger et al., 2015, p. viii). Hence, there is a need to incorporate value-based systems as anti-doping strategies globally.

4.2 A Brief History of Doping

Nolte (2014, p. 82) defines doping as using prohibited substances or methods to enhance sports performance. Doping was a widespread practice characterised by using drugs or other doping substances and methods to improve physical performance in sports. Yesalis and Bahrke (2002, p. 42) argues that doping has been part of the history of human competition. On tracing the historical development of the use of performance-enhancing substances in sports, Yesalis and Bahrke (2002, p. 45) notes that the second half of the nineteenth century witnessed the initial use of modern medicine and a remarkable growth in the use of doping material in their various forms. For Krüger et al.

DOI: 10.4324/9781003370796-5

(2015, p. xviii), the doping systems can be explained and understood only against their background as illegitimate, forbidden methods of performing and winning, which are increasingly becoming popular due to highly sophisticated technological and pharmaceutical products and methods. Krüger et al. (ibid) further argues that doping can be rightly defined by its moral and public condemnation and criminalisation through written rules and laws in the statutes of the sports federation. Yesalis and Bahrke. (ibid) also cite that the last half of the nineteenth century marked scientific experimentation with the anabolic effects of hormones for performance enhancement in sports. Krüger et al. (2015, p. xxiv) aver that

> The use of stimulants like caffeine, cocaine, alcohol, and strychnine, and also the application of oxygen or certain types of radiation, has been practiced in modern sports from the beginning. Yet their use did not seem to be regarded as a problem, given that there was no critical debate at that time, neither inside the world of sport nor among the public as a whole, neither about the risks for athletes' health nor about violations of the sporting ethos of fair play. These drugs and other means of improving athletic achievement and performance were not forbidden by rules, laws, or even public opinion. Pietri Dorando, for example, was disqualified after his marathon race in London in 1908 not because he used drugs, but because he was physically supported by coaches and friends during the last steps before the finish line. However, he was indeed confused and disorientated, probably because of both exertion and drugs.

Krüger et al. (2015, p. xxiv) further adds that international doping historians generally agree that athletes started to experiment with drugs since the 1930s, and soldiers who participated during the Second World War contributed greatly to the spread of drug use and doping in the 1950s. As such these years chiefly contributed to the rise and development of the misuse of new types of drugs in sports, mainly stimulants such as amphetamines. The importance of understanding the general history of drug abuse and other performance-enhancing methods in sport can never be underestimated since it helps one to understand the process of doping initiation through drugs or other methods, addiction and recovery through the application of anti-doping mechanisms.

Therefore, studying a brief history of doping is very relevant to this chapter as supported by Dimeo (2007, p. xi) who strongly emphasises the great need to know where doping came from and why people devoted their time to formulate anti-doping strategies. For Dimeo (ibid), a historical narrative is important for the present times as it will help people to comprehend the predicaments of the current debates and direct them into the future. However, for Krüger et al. (2015, p. xviii), it is very difficult to perceive the history of doping and evaluate it as it really was due to the fact that the development of the doping practice is largely known through anti-doping. Dimeo (2007, p. x) concurs that most historical narratives on doping and anti-doping prove to be frustrating accounts as they fall short in meeting even the fundamental requirements of a good historiography. He (ibid) further argues that these historical narratives were grounded on historically invented stories to prove present relevance and were also not empirically verified. As such these and other factors account for a thin historical narrative on doping.

On the origins of doping, Dimeo (2007, p. xi) rejects the view that the use of performance-enhancing substances in sport originated from professionalism, sports medicine, or athletes' undying desire to win. The motivating force for subscribing to this radical position is the view that, "such one-dimensional explanations avoid the complexities of the changing situations and shifting meanings around drug use in sport. They also avoid a proper assessment of the links between scientific innovation and sports performance" (Dimeo, 2007, p. x). According to Dimeo (2007, p. 3), 1876 marked the beginning of the history of doping in sport through the discovery of the properties of South American coca leave. Rabinbach (1992, p. 22) as cited in Dimeo (2007) substantiates the point that this initiative resulted in the growing interest in finding drugs that would relieve fatigue in workers, athletes, soldiers, and the general population.

4.3 Interconnectedness: The Value of Enhancing Collective Efforts against Doping

The value of interconnectedness is one of the most profound of Ubuntu/Hunhu ethics. Ubuntu is an ethical ideal that is "cooked or brewed in an African pot" (Fiedler et al., 1997; Orobator, 2008). The ethics of Ubuntu reflect on the human relationship with others, which is a relationship that highlights the interconnectedness of all humans, and that this interconnectedness is needed for individuals' self-realisation. In other words, a person is not complete without others (Okyere-Manu and Morgan, 2022, p. 28). It is a submission of this chapter that Ubuntu ethics offers a practical and relevant approach for coming up with an effective anti-doping strategy not only for Africa but also for the international community. This section demonstrates how the Ubuntu value of interconnectedness exhibits communalistic values which manifest themselves even in the sporting fraternity. These values are contrary to individualistic tendencies and can be appropriated and relevantly deployed in the fight against doping and all associated effects. According to Chuwa (2014, p. 12), the principles of Ubuntu present a communal mindset for ethical decisions whereby individuals, community, and the world are connected together. Venter (2004, p. 200) shares the same sentiment that according to the culture of Ubuntu an ideal life results from harmonious relationships among individuals, between individuals and the society. The world of sport is not an exception; it can undoubtedly benefit from the ethics of Ubuntu through the application of principles like interconnectedness.

According to Dimeo (2007, p. 13), doping in all its forms can be rightly regarded as cheating which has negative physical and moral implications. Research evidence shows that doping thrives on the interconnectedness of the factors such as social structures, cultural values, sport federation policies, and the individual athlete's choices, among others. Hence, doping becomes a community problem and not just an individual choice. The nature of doping as a community-shared problem means that the solution should also be community-based and take pride in the value of interconnectedness. Dimeo (2007, p. 15) shares the view that the ideals of sport are a cultural and a social product. He further argues that doping was part of a social history of the development of scientific knowledge which does not exist in a social vacuum. Similarly, Peter Bowler and Iwan Morus (2005, p. 16) contend that science is a human activity which can be heavily influenced by philosophical inquiry, religious beliefs, and political values and professional interests. All these points show that doping thrives on the interconnectedness of different entities, which implies also that anti-doping strategies can be a result of various efforts of connected individuals and community entities. In this regard, Dimeo (2007, p. 6) developed an argument that anti-doping was about social power and was based on Eurocentric religious morality. This chapter also argues that anti-doping strategies can be formulated by incorporating African ethics of Ubuntu/Hunhu that is taking into cognisance various social dimensions embedded in the African ethos. There is no doubt that sport thrives on the web of interconnectedness of human relationships as exhibited by how the sport federation, parents of the athletes, sports administrators, schools, sports clubs, medical practitioners, and other various stakeholders work hand in glove to achieve one goal. Hence, the Ubuntu value of interconnectedness can be harnessed as an effective strategy against doping. This is only achieved through admitting the fact that doping is a socially complex issue and sport is also a social phenomenon that should be addressed effectively through engaging various stakeholders.

4.4 Responsibility as an Anti-Doping Ethical Value

As Chuwa has argued (2014, p. 34), "Responsible human relationships is at the core of ubuntu ethics". It cannot be denied that sport is a field which requires the Ubuntu value of responsibility for its flourishment. As such the value of responsibility becomes key in compelling all concerned stakeholders in sport to be responsible for their actions in a bid to formulate an effective anti-doping strategy. Doping is a cancer which affects physical, moral, and social well-being of the society. In this ethical connection, Mbombo as cited in Chuwa (2014, p. 29) elaborates that whenever a member of a society fell ill, a representative group would accompany the patient to receive medical attention and that sick members of the accompanying group would also be helped without asking for it. All these activities for Chuwa (2014, p. 29) confirm that the healing process in Ubuntu ethics is communitarian, since the whole community of persons is involved and no treatment of any two persons is alike, even if they have the same complaint. The nature of how Africans held their health issues means that all the members of the community, the sick and the non-sick, would become responsible for their fellow human beings. As such the war on doping automatically becomes the responsibility of the society and not just an individual athlete war.

Ubuntu healthcare addresses not only the visible symptoms, but the possible underlying physiogenic, psychological, social, and ontological causes. Healing is a process of reconciliation. Healing reconciles and restores the lost unity within the self, between the self and the society, between the self and the diseased, between the self and the cosmos, and between the self and God. Ubuntu perspective on human disease and healing is comprehensive and holistic (Chuwa, 2014, p. 40). The ethics of Ubuntu underscores the importance of communal existence and a consciousness of the fact that we all have a responsibility to ourselves as human beings and also to our environment.

4.5 Ubuntu and Moral Development

To fully appreciate how Ubuntu can be of immense contribution as an anti-doping strategy, let's consider an Ubuntu perspective of moral development. From an Ubuntu perspective moral development is a societal aspect. It takes a society to raise a child and initiate the child into the community. In Mbiti's words, "nature brings the child into the world, but society creates the child into a social being, a corporate person" (Mbiti, 1990, p. 36). For an anti-doping strategy to yield results it must incorporate the society as it is key in the moral development of individuals. Athletes, coaches, physicians, and other stakeholders in sporting hail from the society, so it is the duty of the society to shape them morally from a tender age so that they become responsible citizens who can manage our sporting disciplines and make a doping-free environment. The society has to be at the centre of formulating anti-doping attitudes as young individuals and athletes develop into mature individuals and grown-ups. For Gyekye (1997, p. 42), a person who fails to grow into relating with other persons in an acceptable way is regarded as inhuman. So, if the society is active in putting in place the right values that discourage cheating and doping, then it will become easy to deal with the scourge of rising doping cases in African sports. Thus, for an anti-doping strategy to be effective the values of Ubuntu have to be inculcated and nurtured into the young and adults.

4.6 Ubuntu Relational Perspective and Wellness

Another important aspect of Ubuntu philosophy that needs to be given adequate attention is the centrality of relations when it comes to the well-being of the individual members of the community. Bujo in Chuwa (2014, p. 34) observes that in African traditional society, disease and illness that befall an individual always indicate that something is wrong in human relationships. So, if disease and illness are an indicator of the nature of relationships, it also points to the importance of relations in fighting doping. The negative impact of doping on health has been well documented. The adverse effect of doping can also best be explained in terms of challenges in human relations from an Ubuntu perspective. When we have athletes suffering from different ailments as a result of doping, it really shows that there is a challenges with human relations. So, a good strategy of dealing with doping that truly encompasses Ubuntu values has to deal with human relations first.

Bujo (1992, p. 42) compares African perspective on the sick person with the modern Western one. He writes, "The patient is not rejected as deviant, as a malingerer or as a marginal character, as is often the case in western medicine, but is integrated fully into the continuing concerns of the community." Health care in Ubuntu culture is therefore not only comprehensive and holistic, it is always communitarian. As Chuwa (2014, p. 74) argues, in Ubuntu culture the sick and the people with disabilities are always a responsibility of the society. It remains a responsibility of the African societies to assist athletes who would have been caught up in the scourge to rehabilitate and cope with the effects of doping.

4.7 African Communitarianism

The communitarian nature of Ubuntu ethics plays a significant role in building communities in comparison to that of individuals in any particular ethical situation (Chuwa, 2014, p. 38). Dickson (1977, p. 52) reiterates that communalism is a characteristic feature that defines "Africanness". The personal life is the communal life and the communal life is the personal life. One cannot be without the other. An individual that tries to live outside his community will be like a fish cast out of water onto a dry sandy beach, panting (Chuwa, 2014, p. 72). The role of community in Ubuntu ethics is based on the premise that none of the community members would be what he or she is without the community. Chuwa (2014, p. 74) commented that due to the importance of "otherness" in self-recognition, self-actualisation, and moral development, human relationship is vital in the culture of Ubuntu.

Traditional African life was, and very much still is, community-based: it moves from the community and revolves around the community. A man's achievement depends primarily on how much of his community's standards he accommodates. To exist is to exist in a group. To a large extent, the individual in an African society is subsumed within the requirements of his community and he more or less acts out his community's scripts (Ogbujah, 2007, p. 38).

4.8 Reciprocity between Individual and Community

Another interesting dimension of Ubuntu ethics is the relation between an individual and the community one hails from. Individual athletes, coaches, physicians, and all other stakeholders in sport are members of a community and therefore there should be a reciprocity between them and the society. According to Chuwa (2014, p. 40), the ethics of Ubuntu rests on the assumption that as one is enabled by the community to find oneself and grow as a human person, one should use one's potential for the good of the community. Sporting is enabled by the community in which it takes place, so it is important that sporting personalities are equipped with the values of reciprocity so that they could understand that they are supposed to do good for the community. Obviously, doping is in a way a harm to the very community which would have enabled these sporting personalities to realise their potential. As rightly noted by Chuwa, morality is about human relationships, while a human relationship is about reciprocity. Wrongdoing separates people, disturbs harmony, and is against life. In the same vein, doping separates people and disturbs harmony and is also a threat to the lives of athletes.

4.9 Competition in the Communal Context

At the heart of sporting activities is the issue of competition. Sporting is all about competition but it seems the idea of competition is directly associated with doping. As such there is a need to properly understand the notion of competition from an Ubuntu perspective, especially from a communal perspective. According to Ramose (1999, p. 56), competitiveness is the dogma of economic globalisation. According to this dogma, even the human right to life – human dignity – must be subordinated and reduced to the totalising drive to make profit without limits. Such an understanding and conception of competition is against the spirit and values of Ubuntu. Competition has to be done with limits, especially when it tends to disturb the communal nature of Ubuntu ethics. Even in a competition people should simply accept losing in dignity not to win at any cost, especially those who are tempted to resort to doping. Athletes and all stakeholders in sport need to be properly oriented and grounded in the spirit of sport as espoused by the Ubuntu philosophy of communalism.

4.10 Individual Athletes and Doping

Efforts to curb doping have largely revolved around the athletes as they are the ones who are mostly caught up in doping and they normally shoulder the blame. But what is critical is to focus on the athletes and have the right strategy to equip them with the right values to overcome the temptations of engaging in doping activities. The practice of assigning responsibility for doping behaviour has chiefly been individual-based, focusing mainly on the individual athlete's doping behaviour (Atry, 2013). The individual athletes need to be grounded in the communal values of Ubuntu. Athletes need to appreciate the power dynamics between the individual and the community in the African value system. As pointed out by Ogbujah (2007, p. 21), "the mark of a true African is his ability to put communal interests over and above his individual interests". The African cooperative community spirit goes a long way in portraying altruism: community interests come before personal interests, as the power of the community is superior over that of an individual. Doping is an act of selfishness which does not consider the common good but rather focuses on individual interest. To succeed in the fight against doping, an anti-doping strategy has to equip individuals with a sense of communalism which helps them to subside personal interests and subordinate themselves to the common good. In that way the ethics of Ubuntu plays a pivotal role in addressing the problem of doping in African sports.

4.11 Coaches' Involvement in Doping and Anti-Doping

Studies on doping have also revealed that it is not athletes who are solely responsible for doping in sport but coaches have also been singled out as being responsible in a number of cases. So, in addressing the doping pandemic, it is also imperative to include these categories as part of the broader strategy.. As such coaches also need to be grounded in the values of Ubuntu. In fact, coaches carry a higher responsibility as they are in charge of the situation as they can easily encourage or discourage the athletes to engage in doping activities.

4.12 Medical Professionals and Doping

Medical professionals by virtue of their professional status carry a much higher obligation to alleviate the doping challenge. But due to the lack of professionalism or lack of grounding in the basic tenets of Ubuntu they have been fingered in a number of cases as being responsible. Yesalis and Bahrke (2002, p. 57) noted that hundreds of physicians and scientists, including top-ranking professors, performed doping research and administered prescription drugs as well as unapproved experimental drug preparations. In the Tour de France doping scandal, it was physicians who served as the primary source of anabolic steroids for over one-third of the steroid users. Athletes can gain access to prohibited medicines from physicians, pharmacists, retail outlets, health and lifestyle magazines, gymnasiums, coaches, family members, fellow athletes, the internet, and the black market (Atry, 2013, p. 20).

4.13 Society and Parental Pressure and Doping

The broader society also has a part to play in the rise of doping in sport. Athletes end up being under pressure to win as a result of the unrealistic expectations from those who surround them. From the immediate family members, the fans, and even the government, pressure mounts on the athlete to win accolades. Yesalis (2002, p. 47) pointed out that an investigation of doping in Olympic sport again concluded that in the rush for gold, governments, coaches, or trainers have often turned a blind eye or have actively supported the use of performance-enhancing substances. The society as a whole needs to revisit the philosophy of Ubuntu and realise that the individual is a congenitally communitarian incapable of existing and really unthinkable except in the complex of relations of the community (Okere, 1996, p. 27).

4.14 Sports Association

Sports governing associations have also not been spared in doping activities. Sporting associations have also been noted to be avoiding taking out dirty linen in public. Yesalis (2002, p. 68) highlighted that sport federations for decades covered up the doping problem, conveniently looking away or instituted drug-testing programmes that were designed to fail. Such a practice might seem to be prudent and the right thing to do in the short run but in the long term it tends to jeopardise all the efforts to fight doping in sports as it tends to appear as a promotion of the act itself.

4.15 Conclusion

This chapter has explored the essence of Ubuntu ethics by showing how it can be effectively applied as an effective anti-doping strategy. Indeed, for any anti-doping strategy to be effective, it has to be inclusive and should incorporate various interest groups. Doping should be treated as a societal challenge not just as a sporting problem. As Boje stated that over 60 years ago, it is our society that emphasises and rewards speed, strength, size, aggression, and, above all, winning. As with other types of drug abuse, doping in sport is primarily a demand-driven problem. In this instance, demand encompasses more than the demand for performance-enhancing drugs by athletes and includes the demand by the fan for the high-level performances that doping brings (Yesalis, 2002, p. 47). Ubuntu as a communal ethics approach becomes an effective approach in efforts to combat doping. This chapter has demonstrated the relevance of Ubuntu as a value system that can be harnessed, revisited, and applied in the quest to deal with doping in sporting and the approach can be useful not only in Africa but also beyond. Ubuntu philosophy emphasises the centrality of the community in addressing societal problems, not in finding individual piecemeal solution. Knowledge about and the inclusion of these sociocultural elements could act as a recipe for the successful implementation of an African ethic that can provide solutions to the problems that the world is grappling with today.

References

Atry, A. (2013). *Transforming the Doping Culture, Whose Responsibility, What Responsibility?* (Doctoral Thesis). Uppsala University.

Bowler, P. J., and Morus, I. R. (2005). *Making Morden Science: A Historical Survey*. Chicago: University of Chicago Press.

Bujo, B. (1992). *African Theology in Its Social Context*. Nairobi and New York: St. Paul Publications/Orbis Books.

Chuwa, L. T. (2014). *African Indigenous Ethics in Global Bioethics*. New York and London: Springer.

Dickson, A. K. (1977). *Aspects of Religion and Life in Africa*. Accra: Ghana Academy of Arts and Sciences.

Dimeo, P. (2007). *A History of Drug Use in Sport 1876–1976: Beyond Good and Evil*. London and New York: Routledge.

Fiedler, K., Gundani, P., and Mijoga, H. (Eds.) (1997). *Theology Cooked in an African Pot*. Zomba-Malawi: Kachere Series.

Gyekye, K. (1997). *Tradition and Modernity: Philosophical Reflections on the African Experience*. New York and Oxford: Oxford University Press.

Krüger, M. Becker, C., and Nielsen, S. (2015*). German Sports, Doping and Politics: A History of Performance Enhancement*. New York: Rowman & Littlefield.

Mbiti, J. S. (1990). *African Religions and Philosophies*. New Hampshire: Heinemann.

Nolte, K. S. (2014). *Doping in Sport: Attitudes, Beliefs and Knowledge of Competitive High School Athletes in Gauteng Province (Vol. 3)*. Doi: 10.7196/SAJSM.542

Ogbujah, C. (2007). "The Individual in African Communalism." *International Journal for Philosophy of Religion*, *23*(1), 13–27.

Okere, T. (Ed). (1996). *Identity and Change*. Washington, DC: The Council for Research in Values and Philosophy.

Okyere-Manu, B., and Morgan, S. N. (2022). "Exploring the Ethics of Ubuntu in the Era of COVID-19." In F. Sibanda (Ed.), *Religion and the COVID-19 Pandemic in Southern Africa*. London: Routledge.

Orobator, A. E. (2008). *Theology Brewed in an African Pot: An Introduction to Christian Doctrine from an African Perspective*. Nairobi: Paulines Publications Africa.

Rabinbach, A. (1992). *The Human Motor Energy, Fatigue, and the Origins of Modernity*. Berkeley: University of California Press.

Ramose, M. (1999). *African Philosophy Through Ubuntu*. Harare, IN: Mond Books.

Venter, E. (2004). The Notion of Ubuntu and Communalism in African Educational Discourse. *Studies in Philosophy and Education, 23*, 149–160. https://doi.org/10.1023/B:SPED.0000024428.29295.03

Yesalis, C., and Bahrke, M. S. (2002). History of Doping in Sport. . *International Sports Studies, 24*(1), 42–76.

Chapter 5

Doping and the African Value System of Ubuntu

Tawanda Mbewe

5.1 Introduction

This chapter critically examines the sociocultural impact of doping on the African value terrain and tradition of Ubuntu. Prospects of financial gains and pressure to win medals and defend some sporting titles have lured some athletes to resort to the unorthodox doping method to excel in some sporting disciplines. This worldwide phenomenon has raised some grave moral concerns. This chapter pays particular attention to how the act of doping impacts African moral values, which are predicated on the ethical concept of Ubuntu. Although doping has become a global challenge, there is minimal research on doping and the African value system. Apart from the avalanche of scholarly works on the causes and effects of doping in professional sport, there has not been much scholarly work on doping and African moral values.

Interestingly, most works on doping in Africa have focused on the moral issues of the act from a Western conception of morality. Little if no attention has been placed on how our African value system is being impacted and, ultimately, how it can contribute to the issue. In discussing African culture and values, we do not presuppose that all African societies have the same explanation(s) for events, the same language, the same mode of dressing, etc. Rather, there are underlying similarities shared by many African societies which, when contrasted with other cultures, reveal a wide gap of difference (Idang, 2015, p. 97). Differences may exist in Africa regarding which course of action to take in a given moral dilemma. However, the African moral conception is premised on advancing the best interests and well-being of the community. The well-being and good of the society are the basis of Ubuntu moral philosophy, so any discussion about African morality must incorporate Ubuntu's place and relevance. Specific forms of behaviours in sporting can be evaluated using this African conception of morality, or a moral assessment can be done to assess their impact on the worldview and ethical grounding of the African people.

DOI: 10.4324/9781003370796-6

5.2 What Is Doping?

The meaning of the word "doping" can be adequately understood in its historical context. So, a brief background of how the term originated would be of value. Rosen (2008, p. viii) traces the origins of the word "doping" to Zulu warriors in South Africa who used an alcoholic extract of grape skins that the Afrikaans settlers called "dope" to increase their strength and endurance before heading off to battle. By the late nineteenth or early twentieth century, the word was introduced into English as "dope" and "doping". One of the first uses of the word was to describe the act of giving racehorses illegal medications or substances, with the idea of changing (either improving or diminishing, depending on the doper's intentions) the way the horse performed. Today's use of the term implies that the athlete is doing something wrong, that he or she is breaking the rules.

Generally speaking, "doping" refers to the use of illicit substances and methods by athletes in order to improve athletic performance. According to Atry (2013, p. 11), "there are many ways to enhance athletic performance; some of which are permitted (e.g. training, diet) and some are prohibited (e.g. growth hormones) by sports' governing bodies". Doping involves the use of those prohibited substances in sporting.

According to the International Olympic Committee, doping is any substance or process that can artificially increase work capacity, and which is contrary to sports ethics, as well as the physical and mental integrity of athletes. Robert Alexandru Vlad et al. (2018) maintains that

> for a substance or performance improvement method to be classified as doping, it must meet at least two of the following three criteria: to improve performance, to present a hazard to the health of the athlete and to violate the spirit of sport.
>
> (pp. 530–531)

Let's briefly consider the three elements that are key to an understanding and definition of doping.

Firstly, doping is commonly associated with performance improvement or performance enhancement. Over the last 50 years, public attitude towards professional athletes' use of such drugs has changed from "whatever they need to do their jobs" to disdain and disapproval (Rosen, 2008, p. 40). The idea of performance enhancement can be traced back even to the ancient Greek period, so it's not something new but what has basically changed is the attitude towards it. Over the years attitude towards the act has drastically changed from something that was not a big issue to something that is now disapproved of. So, the use of drugs and substances to enhance performance in sporting has become something unacceptable.

Secondly, doping has also been defined in terms of how it impacts people's health. The fact is that doping has been vehemently condemned in many circles due to its effects on the health of the athletes. Studies on doping have revealed that athletes are able to cross any limit to win in competitions, even if their health is in question (Mahendru et al., 2019). A number of athletes have lost their lives as a result of substance abuse whilst a great number have been adversely affected health-wise and are still struggling with the health effects of some of these banned substances. So, doping encompasses the use of drugs and substances that negatively affect the health of athletes.

Lastly, the other premise that has been part of the definition of doping is its association with a violation of the spirit of sport. The idea of the spirit of sport is all about the core values that define sporting activities, such as fairness and honesty. Doping has been characterised as an activity that violates the spirit of sporting by giving some athletes an unfair advantage over others. The unfair advantage gained as a result of doping has been associated with the violation of the spirit of sporting.

Doping activities have been a common feature in a number of sporting activities. Sports in which the greatest number of violations were recorded are bodybuilding (266 cases) followed by athletics (242) and cycling (218). Football (78) and rugby (54) come 6th and 8th, respectively (Brussels Times, 2019). From the list one can notice that doping is more common in sporting activities that are much more physical in nature. Athletes in such sporting activities are usually tempted to take some performance-enhancing substances so that they can perform better than other athletes.

5.3 Doping in Africa

On the 14th of October in 2017, African news carried a headline titled "Eritrean athlete stripped of titles, banned after failing doping test" (Akwei, 2017, p. 56). That was a sad headline as far as the African story about doping is concerned. According to the publication, the Eritrean world distance mountain runner and champion Petro Mamu was banned for nine months and stripped of his titles after testing positive for doping after two world championships he won in July in Premana, Italy. This is one among some of the unfortunate incidents in which Africans have been caught on the wrong side of doping. Inasmuch as doping has not been as prevalent in Africa as it is in countries in the global north, it is a phenomenon that is steadily creeping in our beloved continent. The steady rise in doping cases is attributed to a number of factors.

Bale and Sang (2014, p. 13) have noted that Western forms of sport were introduced to Africans as a form of social control in colonial contexts, but with the passage of time these sports have become a source of national identity and prestige. Ethiopia, Kenya, and other West African countries, for instance, have now come to be associated with long-distance runners. South Africa is now regarded as a rugby nation. So, inasmuch as most Western sporting disciplines were introduced by former colonial masters for social control, they have later turned out to be sources of national pride and that has had an effect of exerting some form of pressure on the athletes as they suddenly need to be fighting for a national cause. This has led some athletes to turn to doping as a way of winning and defending titles for the sake of their nation's pride. Another factor that has contributed to the rise in doping cases in Africa has been the migration of African athletes to overseas nations. The migration of athletes has been referred to as the new scramble for Africa.

Generally, the term "scramble" for Africa was initially associated with the partition and colonisation of African countries, but it has now assumed a different meaning in sporting activities. The term is now associated with the migration of African athletes to the Global North where they are offered some scholarships or better financial offers. As these athletes migrate to the north they are exposed to a variety of drugs and some end up being tempted to use them for a number of reasons. When these athletes come back home, they are bound to expose those back home to doping and this explains why doping is slowly creeping into African sport. For Mbih (2015, p. 4), age-cheating is for African football what doping is for European and American sports. His argument is that in African sports the disease is not doping; it is age-cheating.

Inasmuch as Mbih argues that doping is not much of a problem in Africa so far, we need to be wary even of those few cases that have been identified in Africa. In fact, it is a prudent idea to be on the lookout even if the cases are still few so as to avoid their proliferation like in the global north. However, the low numbers might suggest that either doping is not a widespread problem or that the testing facilities/ level of testing in Africa is not at the scale of Western countries. Performance enhancement techniques have become more and more sophisticated and, at the same time, increasingly more difficult to detect (Rosen, 2008, p. 112). So, at the moment it is very difficult to tell or measure the actual numbers as we currently do not have the necessary testing apparatus at our disposal in Africa.

According to the latest rankings by the World Anti-Doping Agency (WADA), South Africa was in the top 10, signalling the fact that doping is now an African problem and not just a European one (The Brussels Times, 2019). According to the South African Institute for Drug-Free Sport's (2022) chief executive Khalid Galant, there have not been significant doping problems with "minority" sports in South Africa because the financial rewards in these sports were not substantial. There tends to be a strong correlation between financial rewards and the potential for doping. Sporting activities with good financial rewards have generally tempted athletes to engage in doping activities. Inasmuch as there are many other factors that contribute to doping, the main ones have been noted to be financial rewards and pressure to win and defend titles.

5.4 Doping and Social and Cultural Setting

Tahiraj and Hakaj (2021, p. 531) contend that the sociocultural environment in which athletes find themselves, live, and train determines their attitude towards doping. So, a fair assessment of doping in Africa should also consider the African social and cultural terrain which is hugely premised on Ubuntu. Ubuntu philosophy best explains how Africans respond to doping and its effects. The African cultural and social environment can partly explain how African athletes have generally responded to doping activities and how doping is not as prevalent as it is in other continents. But it remains a fact that doping is slowly creeping in and this can be explained in terms of how some Africans are slowly moving away from their cultural and ethical foundations which define their identity as Africans. Doping has been rife in Europe partly because of their value system which is premised on individual liberty and freedom.

5.5 Philosophy of Ubuntu

According to Lefa (2015, p. 51), Ubuntu lies at the heart of the African way of life and impacts every aspect of people's well-being. Thus, the present effort seeks to consider people's well-being in sporting activities. Ubuntu is an African philosophy that places emphasis on "being human through other people" (Mugumbate, 2013, p. 83). It is Africa's worldview of societal relations. It is a social and humanistic ethic. Ubuntu philosophy is integrated into all aspects of day-to-day life throughout Africa and is a concept shared by all tribes in Southern, Central, West, and East Africa among people of Bantu origin (Rwelamila, Talukhaba, and Ngowi, 1999, p. 338). Ubuntu is the basis of African communal cultural life. It expresses the interconnectedness, common humanity, and the responsibility of individuals to each other (Koster, 1996, pp. 99–118; Nussbaum, 2003, pp. 21–26). The culture of Ubuntu presents a communal mindset for ethical decisions whereby individuals, community, and the world are connected together (Chuwa, 2012, p. 76). It is the submission of this chapter to argue that the values and ethos behind Ubuntu should also be displayed by Africans in sporting activities and this can go a long way in eradicating the problem of doping in sport. Ubuntu philosophy therefore underpins any grouping within an African society.

5.6 Ethics in Sport

Sporting like any human activity has to be guided by a set of moral principles. Special rules and laws that govern specific sporting disciplines are not adequate to regulate sports persons and they cannot relegate the place and relevance of ethics in sporting. Ethics goes beyond sports rules and regulations. Uzor and Ujuagu (2021) pointed out that the commercialisation of contemporary sport has made winning the goal of every athlete. Even if winning has become the number one priority in sporting, it must not come at the expense of our moral values. Sporting has to be subjected to our everyday moral norms as a people unless we do not consider sporting to be part of our everyday lives. In the same manner we also need to situate Ubuntu in the whole sporting matrix. Africans as a people are not supposed to lose their Ubuntu moral compass and ethical guiding principles. Doping is one of those instances where African sports personalities should cherish and value the place of Ubuntu in their sporting activities. The value and place of ethics in sport can be noted in the following propositions:

1 Ethics as an integral component of sporting activities. Ethics is an important component of any sporting discipline as any inadequate consideration of the relevance of ethics can turn any sporting discipline into an undesirable one.
2 Ethics as a lubricant. Ethics as a lubricant is there to avoid friction between the parties involved in sporting activities.
3 Ethics as an adhesive. As an adhesive ethics in sports helps to create bond and relationships between different nationalities. Sports have great potential for bringing together even warring parties. Ethics in sport can actualise the potential that sports have.

The Spirit of Sport and the Spirit of Ubuntu

Many a times people speak about the spirit of sport without elaborating what it entails. The phrase has become popular when people talk about the need to uphold certain minimum moral benchmarks in sports.

The spirit of sport basically refers to the purpose of engaging in sporting activities and it also incorporates the values that are associated with sporting activities. On the other hand, the spirit of Ubuntu considers human action to be social (Chuwa, 2012, p. 65).

There are some striking similarities between the spirit of sport and the spirit of Ubuntu – hence the need to examine how the two relate and how both are impacted by doping. For Schneider and Friedman (2006, p. 15), "doping represents a perversion of sports. It converts the beauty of sport, the glory of striving and achieving and outdoing physical limitations into mere biotechnology". It can be argued that the spirit of sport enshrines values that are embodied in the spirit of Ubuntu. Doping has been characterised as something that is "fundamentally contrary to the spirit of sport". WADA (2009, p. 14) characterises the "spirit" of sport through values such as ethics, fair play, and honesty; respect for rules and laws; respect for self and other participants; and excellence in performance. Values such as fairness and honesty are at the heart of Ubuntu ethics, which is to say the spirit of Ubuntu truly shares a lot in common with the spirit of sport. Both aim at achieving the promotion of the interests of all concerned members.

Doping and the Common Good

The ethics of Ubuntu are premised on furthering and promoting the good in a society and this entails the avoidance of that which brings harm. The same applies to sporting activities as they are intended to entertain, recreate and contribute to the overall good of the society. Of course, sport can also lead to some ills here and there depending on the nature and the circumstances surrounding the sporting event. Ubuntu ethics is all about what furthers the interests of the community and the society and the assumption is that the good for the society would also cascade to the good of the individual members. Chuwa (2012, p. 65) notes that "Ubuntu ethics considers any human act which ignores the common good to be unethical on the grounds that personhood is facilitated by, and dependent on, human society". As has been noted earlier, doping has a number of negative effects from the individual to the community. The negative effects range from health challenges to threatening the well-being of the community itself. So, doping can be regarded as something that seriously poses a threat to the well-being of the community. Doping does not only affect the individual athletes concerned but it has also serious moral concerns to the community as a whole. It even goes against the whole idea of sporting in a community. Instead of having sport as something that binds the community, doping frustrates the Ubuntu spirit and the ethos of sport, thereby spreading a divisive miasma in societies and communities. Ubuntu ethics is all about celebrating and cherishing values that work on building the community, values that encourage and promote human flourishing. That is the core of both sports ethos and the ethics of Ubuntu, which doping compromises and undermines.

Doping and Individual Autonomy

One of the arguments that has been raised in defence of doping activities is the fact that individuals should be allowed to freely choose what's good for them. The whole idea of autonomy is closely associated with the idea of freedom and individual liberty. It is important to analyse the idea of individual liberty from an African understanding so that we can demonstrate why the idea raises challenges in Africa. Ansah and Mensah (2018, p. 16) rightly noted that early communitarian scholars who only emphasised the supremacy of the community without recourse to the individual's individuality and the rights that come with it are categorised as radical communitarians, proponents of which are John Mbiti, Ifeanyi Menkiti, Alasdair Macintyre, Charles Taylor, and others. According to Senghor's views, solidarity should take precedence over individual decision and activity. Community needs should be precedent to individual needs. He contends that Africans place more emphasis on the "communion of persons than on their autonomy" (Chuwa, 2012, p. 77). So, inasmuch as Africans do not totally reject the idea of individual autonomy, they place more emphasis on the communion of persons in the words of Senghor. Unlike radical communitarianism that denies liberalism, moderate communitarianism shows that individual rights, and by extension individuality, are recognised in a communitarian framework. Gykeye argues for moderate communitarianism as it accords equal moral status to both the community and the individual.

Ntibagirirwa (1999, p. 24) states that Ubuntu arms one with "normative principles for responsible decision-making and action, for oneself and for the good of the whole community. The idea of autonomy, though a noble one, must only be understood in the context of the good of the whole community. So, in this regard we cannot defend doping on the grounds of individual autonomy as this is against the principles of Ubuntu ethics which place emphasis on the community and not on individuals. Thus, it is not to say that individuals are not important but again their importance is manifested in the societal context. Freedom in particular and virtue in general, therefore, are contingent on and defined by community, society, and the common good. No individual is greater than the society; individual members of the society are parts of, and enabled by the society (Chuwa, 2012).

By engaging in doping, one is merely trying to be greater than the other participants in the sporting community and ultimately in the entire community. Thus, the idea of individual liberty and freedom has to be properly understood in the context of the community and not merely in individual members. As such doping negatively impacts the societal values and it tends to be premised on the importance of the individual athlete at the expense of the other athletes.

Doping as a Form of Cheating

There is no doubt that doping as an attempt to win in games through the use of unorthodox means is a form of cheating. Doping, as a form of cheating, can be understood in terms of gaining advantage over one's opponent in an unfair manner, or, alternatively, affecting the results of the competition in ways that are unfair (Atry, 2013, p. 23). Cheating by its own nature is a wanton disregard of the value of relations. Sport is inherently a rule-driven enterprise (Schneider and Friedman, 2006). This makes it something contrary to the ideals and values of Ubuntu.

Thaddeus Metz (2007, p. 325) identified a concise ethical principle based on African relationality, solidarity, and reciprocity: "an act is right just insofar as it is a way of living harmoniously or prizing communal relationships, ones in which people identify with each other and exhibit solidarity with one another; otherwise, an act is wrong". For Metz, doping is a form of cheating that is contrary to the ideals of solidarity and reciprocity. So, cheating is wrong from an African perspective as it violates the principle of solidarity which is a key component of Ubuntu ethics. African athletes should be groomed and nurtured along the values of Ubuntu as it is the key for sustaining human relations.

As correctly noted by Tutu in Battle (1997, p. 66), a person who embraces Ubuntu is

> open and available to others, affirming of others, does not feel threatened that others are able and good, for he or she has a proper self-assurance that comes from knowing that he or she belongs to a greater whole and is diminished when others are humiliated or diminished, when others are tortured or oppressed.

Doping is an acknowledgement of the fact that one is insecure and not comfortable with their capabilities, so they resort to cheating as a way of making up for their deficiencies. It's a sign of being threatened by the ability of other athletes. Cheating is one of the vices that impedes social and ethical growth in a society. Cheating in sporting activities naturally extends to other facets of human life. It threatens the moral fibre of the African community. So, doping has to be fought from all corners if we are to preserve the moral integrity of the African community. Anti-doping efforts should not be seen merely as a sporting issue but a communal one that is contrary to the survival and existence of the community as a whole.

Anti-Doping as a Communal Issue

Effort to curb and combat doping can very much be seen as a way of trying to advance the common good in a society and as a paternalistic stance. Ubuntu ethics as an approach to anti-doping looks at the malpractice from the standpoint of the community and not of sporting personalities who are involved in or are affected by the act. Anti-doping has to be all-encompassing and must be regarded as a communal effort. Ubuntu calls for collective efforts in fighting and curbing societal ills.

In Ubuntu culture, the sick and people with disabilities are always a responsibility of the society (Chuwa, 2012). In the same vein athletes affected or who can be affected by doping become a cause of concern for the whole community. Doping is not an isolated challenge but rather it's the community's responsibility to act against it. Unlike the selfish and egoistic tendencies associated with doping, efforts to combat the vice have to be inclusive. Doping activities work against the common good of the society and thus have the potential to promote values contrary to the values of Ubuntu.

In Gyekye's words, "the preservation of the society's integrity and values enjoins the individual to exercise her rights within limits, transgressing which will end in assaulting the rights of other individual or the basic values of the community" (1997, p. 46) . In this regard athletes are supposed to work so as to preserve social integrity not just to think of personal glory associated with lifting medals. It is every athlete's desire to lift trophies and medal but that has to be done within the confines of ethical and societal values.

The position that doping harms society is based on the fact that doping harms individuals in society, especially children who see athletes as their role models (Schneider and Friedman, 2006, p. 5). Doping activities do not have the effect of harming athletes only but the whole society is endangered. To effectively combat doping any anti-doping strategy and framework must take the collective and inclusive approach to doping. Anti-doping education has to fit into the whole moral education of a community and the nation at large. The school curriculum should also incorporate an anti-doping stance as part of the broad ethical upbringing of learners.

5.7 Conclusion

In this chapter, I have shown that there is a close link between the ethics of Ubuntu and the ethics of sport. Efforts to curb doping in African sporting have to incorporate and appeal to the African spirit of Ubuntu. It is evident that doping contradicts the place and spirit of Ubuntu among Africans. So, any serious strategy of dealing with doping in Africa has to consider its implications for the African ethical and cultural values which are premised on humanness.

Because the causes of doping in Africa involve an interaction of political, economic, social, and cultural factors, the solution to the problem must involve a holistic approach that takes all these interconnected causative factors into account. This must include a paradigm shift in the way in which doping is looked at in Africa. Doping is not only a challenge for those who are into sports but rather it is a communal challenge. Doping issues in Africa have to be looked at using the lenses of the community not just to focus on individual personalities. An Ubuntu-based approach to anti-doping efforts regards doping as a community challenge that must be addressed as such. A revisit to our Ubuntu ethos can help us to refocus our energies and strategies, which is key to combating doping. Sport, as a strong builder for equality, solidarity, and inclusion, especially of the most disadvantaged and vulnerable within African communities, is a foundation for building healthier and peaceful societies in Africa.

References

Akwei, I. (2017). Eritrean Athlete Stripped of Titles, Banned After Failing Doping Test. *Africanews*. Available at www.africanews.com/2017/10/14/eritrean-athlete-stripped-of-titles-banned-after-failing-doping-test//#:~:text=Eritrean%20world%20distance%20mountain%20runner,used%20as%20medication%20for%20Asthma.

Ansah, R., and Mensah, M. (2018). Gyekye's Moderate Communitarianism: A Case of Radical Communitarianism in Disguise. *OGIRISI: A New Journal of African Studies, 19*(2), 1–26. http://dx.doi.org/10.4314/og.v15i1.1

Atry, A. (2013). *Transforming the Culture of Doping: Whose Responsibility, What Responsibility?* (Doctoral Thesis). Uppsala University.

Bale, J., and Sang, J. (2014). Kenyan Running Movement Culture, Geography and Global Change. London: Routledge.

Battle, M. (1997). *The Ubuntu Theology of Bishop Desmond Tutu*. Pilgrim's Press.

Chuwa, L. T. (2012). *African Indigenous Ethics in Global Bioethics*. Springer.

Gyekye, K. (1997). *Tradition and Modernity: Philosophical Reflections on the African Experience*. Oxford University Press.

Idang, G. E. (2015). African culture and values. *Phronimon, 16*(2), 97–111.

Koster, J. D. (1996). Managing the Transformation. In K. Bekker (Ed.), *Citizen Participation in Local Government* (pp. 99–118). Van Schaik.

Lefa, B. J. (2015). Ubuntu in South African Education. *Studies in Philosophy and Education, 1*(10), 4–15.

Mahendru, D., Kumar, S., Prakash, A., and Medhi, B. (2019). Drugs in Sport: The Curse of Doping and Role of Pharmacologist. *Indian Journal of Pharmacology, 51*(1), 1–3.

Mbih, T. (2015). The Ethical and Social Implications of Age-cheating in Africa. *International Journal of Philosophy, 3*(1), 1–1.

Metz, T. (2004). Toward an African Moral Theory. *The Journal of Political Philosophy, 15*(3), 321–344. https://doi.org/10.1111/j.1467-9760.2007.00280.x

Mugumbate, J., and Nyanguru, A. (2013). Exploring African Philosophy: The Value of Ubuntu in Social Work. *Faculty of Social Sciences – Papers, 3266,* 82–100.

Ntibagirirwa, S. (1999). *In a Retrieval of Aristotelian Virtue Ethics in African Social and Political Humanism: A Communitarian Perspective, 104.* University of Natal.

Nussbaum, B. (2003). Ubuntu: Reflections of a South African on our common humanity. *Reflections, 4,* 21–26. https://doi:10.1162/152417303322004175

Rosen, D. M. (2008). *Dope: A History of Performance Enhancement in Sports from the Nineteenth Century to Today*. Praeger.

Rwelamila, P. D., Talukhaba, A. A., and Ngowi, A. B. (1999). Tracing the African Project Failure Syndrome: The Significance of "Ubuntu". *Engineering, Construction and Architectural Management, 6,* 335–346. https://doi.org/10.1046/j.1365-232x.1999.00120.x

Schneider, A. J., and Theodore, F. (2006). *Gene Doping in Sports: The Science and Ethics of Genetically Modified Athletes*. Amsterdam: Elsevier.

South African Institute for Drug Free Sport. (2022). *Doping Not Confined to the "Usual" Suspects*. May 12. http://drugfreesport.org.za/doping-not-confined-to-the-usual-suspects/

Tahiraj, E., and Hakaj, E. (2021). Doping in Sports — Causes and Consequences. *Teaching Methodology and Didactics Physical Education. Croatia, 19,* 531–535.

The Brussels Times (December 21, 2019). *Belgium in Top 10 List of Countries with Most Sports Doping Cases*. Available at www.brusselstimes.com/85118/belgium-in-top-10-list-of-countries-with-most-sports-doping-cases

Uzor, T. N., and Ujuagu, N. (2021). Ethical Issues in Sports: Unfair Advantages Due to Pressure to Win at All Costs. *Journal of Academy of Dental Education, 16*(2), 105–115.

Vlad, R. A., Hancu, G., Popescu, G. C., and Lungu, J. A. (2018). Doping in Sports, a Never-Ending Story? *Advanced Pharmaceutical Bulletin*, *8*(4), 529–534.
WADA (2009). *WADA International Standard for the Prohibited List*. Available at: www.wada-ama.org/rtecontent/document/code_v2009_en.pdf

Chapter 6

African Indigenous Sports Remedies and Doping

Stella Patience Mikwana, Agatha Magombo, Manuel Kasulu, and Yamikani Ndasauka

6.1 Introduction

This chapter explores the use of African indigenous remedies and rituals in sports and how they satisfy the criteria of doping as ascribed by the World Anti-Doping Agency (WADA). The chapter also explores the perceived effectiveness of the said remedies and ritual practices. The chapter argues that some practices in African indigenous knowledge systems in sports embody doping parameters. According to Nolte et al. (2014), doping is the use of prohibited substances and methods in sports. In the World Anti-Doping Code, doping is outlined to be fundamentally contrary to the spirit of sport and the intrinsic value of sports. The spirit of sports is the essence of the Olympics and the pursuit of excellence through a person's natural talents (WADA, 2021). For a substance or a performance-enhancing method to be considered doping, it must at least satisfy two of the following three criteria: to improve performance, to present a hazard to the health of an athlete, and to violate the spirit of sport (Vlad et al., 2018). The chapter is organised into six sections which include an introduction, WADA's doping criteria and its challenges, an exposition of some African traditional remedies and rituals in sports, an exemplification of the scientific basis of some African indigenous remedies and rituals, and WADA's criteria vis-à-vis African indigenous remedies, which a conclusion will follow.

Although relatively new in Africa, sports governing bodies also promote clean sports by compiling lists and classes of prohibited substances and performance-enhancing methods, many of which are pharmacological. Some of these classes outlined by WADA and the International Medical Committee include stimulants, narcotics, and anabolic agents (MacAuley, 1996; Kicman and Gover, 2003). According to Brian Morris (1989), traditional medicine and ritual practices are part and parcel of indigenous knowledge systems, especially for rural African people. African traditional medicine, rituals, and superstition are essential aspects of African culture, and many people substitute pharmaceutical medicine with traditional medicine. Although not recognised by sports governing bodies, African traditional medicine and

DOI: 10.4324/9781003370796-7

rituals are perceived to give athletes secret power (Mulungwa, 2018). Mpepu, Mangolomela, and Tailsmen are rituals that give people unnatural power and strength; therefore, athletes who partake in such rituals are believed to have a competitive edge over others.

Sports governing bodies are concerned that some athletes use anabolic steroids to improve endurance, muscle strength, and size. In Africa, some people use traditionally produced anabolic substances such as Nganganga and Gondolosi instead of pharmaceutical anabolic substances. In contrast, Chamba (Indian hemp) is believed to be a stimulant and a charm-neutralising agent. As this chapter will argue, the use of these charms and indigenous remedies by African athletes may enhance performance, present hazards to the health of athletes, and goes against the spirit of sports and hence considered doping. Therefore, WADA should aim to find ways of regulating or prohibiting them.

6.2 WADA's Criteria for Prohibiting Substances and Methods

The use of prohibited substances and methods in sports is a recurring global problem that has, in turn, influenced WADA to declare war against doping in sports. According to WADA, doping can be defined as the use of performance-enhancing substances or methods as well as the violation of any of the following anti-doping rules: the presence of a prohibited substance(s) in an athlete's sample, the use or attempted use of a banned substance or method, refusal to submit to sample collection after being notified, failure to submit athlete's whereabouts information and missed tests, tampering with any part of the doping control process, possession of a prohibited substance or method, trafficking a prohibited substance or method, administering or attempting to administer a prohibited substance or method to an athlete, complicity in an anti-doping rule violation, and prohibited association with athlete supporting personnel who have engaged in doping (WADA, 2021).

In the war against doping in sports, WADA has put in place policies and codes regarding prohibited substances and methods. At the core of the guidelines on doping control rest four fundamental principles, namely, the need for sports to set a good example, the necessity to ensure a level playing field, the responsibility to protect the health of the athletes, and the importance of preserving the integrity (spirit) of sport (Smith et al., 2008). In Article 4 of the anti-doping code, WADA outlines the criteria for assigning a substance or method as constituting doping. The standards embody three propositions. Firstly, if the substance or method has the potential to enhance or enhances sports performance. Secondly, if the use of the substance or method poses an actual or potential threat to the athlete's health. Thirdly, if the use of the substance or method violates the integrity (spirit) of sport as determined by

WADA in the World Anti-Doping Code (WADA, 2021). Therefore, a substance or performance-enhancing method is considered doping provided that the said substance or method meets at least two of the three criteria. Additionally, WADA also considers substances or methods that have the potential to mask the use of prohibited substances and methods for the banned substances and methods lists.

The first criterion that WADA considers is whether a substance or method has the potential to improve performance. This includes the use of drugs and techniques that induce strength, mental alertness, and muscle growth, for example, human growth enzymes, gene modification, and sports technologies such as shoes fashioned to imitate the hoofs of a horse so that an athlete would have more leverage. Given that there is relevant evidence to support the claim that a substance or method has the potential to improve performance or improves performance in sports, it is placed on the prohibited list. In so doing, WADA ensures a level playing field for all parties involved in sport. To this effect, WADA has a monitoring programme where all sports bodies under WADA are charged with keeping a close watch on all the substances and methods on the prohibited list (WADA, 2021).

The second criterion that WADA considers is whether a substance or method poses an actual or a potential threat or risk to an athlete's health and general well-being (WADA, 2021). WADA takes its responsibility seriously, looking after the physical and mental well-being of athletes and considering the aspect of human rights. The World Anti-Doping Code makes provision for the use of some drugs on the prohibited list under exceptional circumstances. WADA recognises that performance-enhancing drugs (PEDs) and methods have the potential to alter the human body and its biological functions. Although some medicines and methods can potentially improve or enhance athletic performance, they are extremely dangerous to the health of athletes, and the effects these methods can have on health are both physiological and psychological. For instance, the use of certain drugs can have consequences such as the development of breast tissue in males, liver damage, increased aggressiveness, depression, and impaired memory.

WADA also considers whether a substance or performance-enhancing method violates the spirit of sport. WADA defines the spirit of sport as the intrinsic value of sports, the ethical pursuit of human excellence through dedication, and the perfection of the athlete's natural talents and abilities (WADA, 2021). The integrity of sport consists of respect for rules, other competitors, fair competition, a level playing field, and generally the practice of clean sports. The integrity of sports, according to WADA, is the celebration of the human spirit and mind. Thus, doping is entirely contrary to the preservation of the integrity of sport.

Even though WADA's criteria are widely used by sports governing bodies worldwide, some scholars have argued that the code is based on what can best be described as questionable ethical grounds. According to Kayser and

Mauron (2007), WADA's criteria are vague in that they cannot withstand critical reflection and create more problems than they can solve. In the first place, the involvement of medical professionals in anti-doping efforts goes against the principles of medical ethics with specific reference to non-maleficence and the protection of privacy. Medical professionals working in doping control are placed in ethically tricky positions as they are required to disclose the personal and private information of their clients/patients to officials. In some cases, medical personnel violate the principle of non-maleficence. For example, Aminatou Seyni, Margaret Wambui, Francine Niyonsaba, and Caster Semenya have been barred from partaking in activities of their preference at major sporting events because they have high testosterone levels (Lopez, 2021). Even though testosterone is not a gender-specific hormone, these women have been forced to either chemically or surgically lower the levels of this hormone in their bodies which can potentially harm them by reducing their heart rate (Scientific American, 2019). Even with prior knowledge of this potential harm to the athletes, medical professionals in anti-doping control still prescribe medication to these athletes.

In an interview, Semenya revealed that the medication that she is forced to take made her constantly sick. Additionally, the war against doping is dangerous because it has become an underground practice, making it more difficult for athletes who dope because of the unhygienic conditions in which they are forced to practise doping (Kayser and Mauron, 2007). For instance, athletes may be forced to use unsterilised instruments such as needles or even administer lethal dosages. They argue for medically supervised doping, where athletes would be allowed to dope under the careful supervision of medical professionals. In this case, we assume that Kayser and Mauron were in fact arguing for other forms of doping other than chemical doping because most of them feature on WADA's list. Perhaps other forms of performance enhancements, especially technological, can be considered here, including shoes that are designed like hooves of a horse which give an athlete more leverage and hence increasing speed.

According to Geeraets (2018), WADA's analysis of the third criterion is subjective as it does not clearly explain what "spirit of sport" means. As prescribed by WADA, the third criterion has values that cannot be adequately coordinated simultaneously. At present, the concept of fair play/level playing field fails to consider other sources of inequality among athletes. It is a fact that some people have natural gene mutations that may give them an advantage over other athletes, while others have pharmaceutically mutated genes and body enhancements. The case of a cross-country skier from Finland who had a natural rare gene mutation that enabled him to carry more oxygen in his blood than the average male is a telling case in point (Epstein, 2013). Indeed, he went on to win three medals in the 1963 winter Olympic Games. Arguably, WADA does not consider such inequality when it comes to maintaining a level playing field. Thus, naturally, gene mutations that have a bearing on performance in sports are acceptable inequalities, while pharmaceutically achieved gene mutations are unacceptable (Kayser and Mauron, 2007). However, it is practically impossible for WADA to achieve equality in sports in the manner in which Kayser and company argue. People worldwide are born with different genetic dispositions, and are naturally different in terms of physical attributes such as size and height. Therefore, natural differences cannot be considered an inequality even if particular individuals can benefit from it.

Additionally, the contextual complexities involved in managing the use of drugs in sports make it difficult for people to agree on how best doping can be handled (Smith and Stewart, 2015). They argue that WADA's code has been unable to control doping, and neither has it been able to protect the health of the athletes as some PEDs do not appear on the prohibited list; hence, athletes are free to use these drugs. This is an apparent violation of the concept of a level playing field (Smith and Stewart, 2015).

The current anti-doping policies are problematic and should be productively reviewed. For instance, the World Anti-Doping Code prescribes that for a substance or performance-enhancing method to be considered doping, it must meet at least two of the three criteria in the code. This becomes a problem because WADA to a certain extent implies that it is not a problem if athletes use substances or methods as long as they do not meet the criteria. Consequently, it is not wrong to conclude that there is no hierarchy in WADA's criteria. In addition, Kayser and Smith (2008) argue that the current anti-doping test protocols violate an athlete's privacy excessively and the notion of personal freedom. In this regard, WADA and other sports governing bodies can be afforded leeway in terms of respecting the personal freedoms of athletes, but they should not be demonstratably excessive.

Some athletes are subjected to degrading physical examinations and endure procedures that can best be described as a violation of their human rights. A good example here is Caster Semenya, a South African athlete who offered to show track officials her body because they would not believe that she was biologically a female. In later years Semenya was forced to take medication to alter her natural hormone levels for her to be able to compete at significant meets, and because of the restrictions placed on her, she was unable to defend her Olympic title in Tokyo. Semenya has a natural condition known as the difference in sex development. The World Athletics Organisation and other sports governing bodies have forced Semenya to take medication to lower her testosterone levels. However, World Athletics has failed to disclose the medication Semenya was placed on and its dosage. In a recent interview with HBO, Semenya admitted that she felt tortured by the entire experience and has lived in constant fear of suffering a heart attack due to the medication she is forced to take (Imray, 2022). The conduct of the various sports governing bodies involved in Semenya's case violated her freedom and privacy. The war on doping should not be based on moral distaste for drugs but on solid and rational grounds. Kayser and Smith (2008) argue that it would be more beneficial for WADA to provide tangible and sufficient evidence of the effects of drug use in sports to help athletes see first-hand what the results of drug use can be, rather than use coercion. In light of this criticism WADA's anti-doping criteria, current policies, and code must be reviewed.

6.3 African Traditional Remedies and Rituals in Sports

Plants/flora products and animals and their products have been used for their medicinal properties for hundreds of years, and the use of plants and animals for medicinal purposes is a widespread practice in the world. However, according to the World Health Organization, these practices vary because of different social and cultural heritages (Sofowora, 1996). In Africa, traditional remedies and rituals are deeply rooted in the African understanding of sickness and disease. Thus, traditional remedies and rituals are part and parcel of African culture and tradition. Traditional healers are crucial in providing traditional remedies and ritual divinations as they take a holistic approach to ailments by treating their patients' spiritual and physical well-being.

In Africa, traditional medicines are used not only in treating illnesses but also in bringing good luck and the general well-being of a person. Many Africans believe that bad luck and sickness result from factors such as witchcraft, ancestral spirits, and evil evoked by people with ill will. This understanding is prevalent in all areas of an African person's life, and only traditional remedies and rituals are reliable in countering such forces (Ngubane, 1977). Even though conventional African treatments and practices lack scientific proof of efficacy, they are used in different areas of life, whether private or social. According to Mulungwa et al. (2018), a range of pharmacological compounds are present in traditional remedies, but it is not known which of the said compounds have therapeutic properties. In 2010, Fédération Internationale de Football Association (FIFA) officials urged WADA to address concerns that World Cup players might attempt to use traditional remedies, therefore gaining an unfair advantage over other players and violating the principle of a level playing field as WADA prescribes (Mcgrath, 2010). For this chapter, traditional remedies and ritual superstitions are divided into two separate categories, one of which involves individual athletes and the other consists of the team as an entity.

In a quest to attain excellence in sports, individuals engage the services of traditional healers/witch doctors where they are given a tattoo(s) on which substances are smeared; sometimes, individuals are assigned different objects to have on their person during each game. This is done with the belief that the spirits evoked in such practices bring good luck to the bearer and ward off evil spirits. One such traditional practice is locally referred to as Mpepu in Malawi. An individual can do Mpepu as a conventional remedy, but it is sometimes passed down in a family's lineage. This practice involves getting a tattoo(s) where a paste made from a combination of traditional substances is smeared on the tattoo, after which incantations are made by the traditional healer/witch doctor to call on the spirits to make the bearers of the tattoo(s) as light as the wind and invisible. The perceived result of this traditional remedy is that it reduces drag force so that one can run twice as fast as the average athlete and without getting fatigued. It is hard to ascertain whether this is a fact because these practices are shrouded in secrecy. However, people believe that this is effective and thus it has been in existence for generations. This means that Mpepu is believed to improve performance and endurance. Similar to Mpepu is Mangolomera, where the same procedure is followed. The perceived effectiveness of this traditional remedy is that the person has unimaginable strength and is guaranteed to succeed at anything. For instance, apart from sports, Mangolomera is also used by other people to improve the art of public speaking. The belief is that as a result of indulging in the remedy, one has a voice that commands authority, thereby gaining people's attention.

Indian hemp is believed to be a stimulant that induces unimaginable strength in the user, and they feel that they can do almost everything. Apart from inducing power, Indian hemp is believed to be a charm-neutralising agent in cases where a team suspects the opposing side of using traditional remedies to improve their odds of winning the game, and they use Indian hemp by smearing it on articles of clothes and boots to erode the effectiveness of the charms. Some players also use traditionally produced substances such as Gongolosi and Nganganga, believing that they have the same effects as pharmacologically produced anabolic substances. These traditional remedies are perceived to increase muscle size as well as improve endurance in the users. Mchape is also one of the traditional remedies used with the belief that it cleanses (detoxes) the body and acts as a substance that can hide the use of any prohibited substance. Further, Moringa Oleifera which is locally known as Moringa is used to treat ailments such as fever and diabetes, apart from which the tree is believed to induce muscle growth, and local people believe that it chases away evil spirits (Sagona et al., 2020).

Teams in African sports also take part in the use of traditional remedies and rituals as these practices are perceived to diminish the opposition's strength, give the athletes secret power, offer the athletes unbeatable stamina, provide protection from evil spirits, and bring good luck to the team (Cocks and Moller, 2002). The use of spells to diminish the opponent's capacity to play effectively by inducing hallucinations is also prevalent. Some teams also go as far as spending nights in graveyards with traditional healers. After that, they ingest concoctions prepared by a traditional healer. Further, incantations are made to the spirits to make the team members invisible to their opponent. In the aftermath of such activity, they are sometimes forbidden to use each other's names while on the field, fearing that the incantations will backfire on them, rendering them powerless against the opposition. It is the case that sometimes players in a team are unaware that team officials might have indulged in traditional remedies or practices on their behalf to improve the odds of success for their teams.

Superstition is also part and parcel of African sport as many athletes and teams believe that to prevail in various disciplines of sport, they must do as well as avoid doing certain things (Bleak and Frederick, 1998). For instance, using separate entrances when getting into the field or making sure that one player gets into the field well after every other person has gone. Other superstitions include urinating on goal posts and washing the face with urine, sprinkling kitchen salt on goal posts, and dumping pig fat on the opposition with the belief that if the opposition had made any incantations and carried charms/talisman with them with the hope of winning, they would be neutralised. For example, in May 2017, four Malawian super league teams were fined by the Football Association of Malawi (FAM) for engaging in rituals during super league games, such as pouring pig fat on a member of the opposing team and urinating on goal posts (Ndovi, 2017). Another example is that of two teams in Tanzania who were fined for similar *Juju* practices. Emmanuel Muga, a BBC correspondent in Dar es Salaam, reported that in a match between Simba and Yanga football teams, the former's players cast an unknown powder on the pitch and broke eggs in a bid to improve odds of winning to which the latter's players reacted by urinating on the pitch to neutralise the *Juju*. Both teams were later fined by the football association. Muga also reported that there had been allegations that the Tanzanian national team had used funds earmarked for the players to solicit the services of a witch doctor (Muga, 2004). Secrecy and superstition also surround traditional African remedies and rituals as revealing details of these practices are believed to neutralise their effectiveness.

Even though some might argue that the inclusion of rituals and superstition is off the mark because it is to a large extent a matter of faith, it is very essential that the argument advanced by this chapter takes rituals and superstitions into careful consideration. This is the case because many of the rituals – if not all rituals – involve concoctions made from different substances, and sometimes rituals involve objects that act as a talisman (may include particular articles of clothing, jewellery, and tattoos), which satisfies WADA's criteria. Again, call it junk science if we can, but the simple fact that people who partake in these ritual superstitions believe that they are effective is enough reason for WADA to critically regulate their employment in sports. In the absence of scientific proof, a person's psychological condition plays a critical role in determining the outcome of any activity they participate. Therefore, partaking in ritual superstitions boosts people's confidence in themselves and the outcome, and it should be considered as doping because other plays might not have the same advantage. According to Gino and Norton (2013), rituals take on various shapes and forms; they are symbolic behaviours that are performed before, during, or after meaningful events in people's lives, and in their ambiguity differ from culture to culture.

Rituals are performed for different reasons ranging from boosting one's confidence, alleviating grief or problems, rainmaking, and for the intent of performing well in competitions. Rituals may be performed in various religious settings, community settings, and sometimes in solitude for an individual's benefit. Current research has demonstrated that even though rituals may seem to be irrational, they work and psychologists have in recent years revealed that rituals have a causal impact on people's feelings, thoughts, and behaviour (Gino and Norton, 2013). Through the various experiments that they conduct, Gino and Norton (2013) conclude that people's confidence in their abilities, effort, and improved performance were enhanced by various ritual superstitions that they subscribe to despite the lack of a direct causal connection between the rituals they performed and the desired outcomes.

6.4 The Scientific Basis of African Indigenous Remedies and Rituals

The World Health Organization's Centre for Health Development defines African traditional medicines as the total of all forms of knowledge and practices that are based on practical experience or observations that are handed down from generation to generation, whether by word of mouth or in writing, which is subsequently used in diagnosis, prevention, and elimination of physical, mental, as well as social imbalance (Richter, 2003). The World Health Organization estimates that 80% of Africa's population use traditional remedies complementary to Western medicine. Additionally, the African understanding of the cause of illness is grounded in the spiritual realm in which traditional medicine practitioners are expected to treat physical and spiritual problems.

Admittedly, even though many traditional African remedies do not have proven scientific evidence of effectiveness or none thereof, these remedies have survived and have been refined over time, and are currently being used. According to Sofowora (1996), the empirical observations made by man over an extended period of time have served as the basis for the production of cosmetics, drugs, and pharmaceuticals until the emergence of modern medicine. Traditional remedies are effective as some have been proven to contain pharmacological compounds similar to those found in pharmaceutical drugs. The only difference being that those used in modern medicine are synthesised and can be detected using standard tests which is not the case with traditional remedies (Yuan et al., 2016). In addition, some pharmaceutical medications/drugs are produced from the same plants/plant species used in traditional remedies. The lack of scientific proof for most herbs/traditional remedies is devastating to the acceptance of its efficacy by practitioners of modern medicine. Furthermore, the occult practices linked to African traditional medicine cannot be scientifically proven; hence, these remedies are regarded with suspicion (Sofowora, 1996). However, traditional African medications are preferred by locals as compared to modern medicine because they are cheap and easily accessible.

For instance, Gondolosi is mainly known as an aphrodisiac as it improves testosterone levels, enlarges male genitalia, and induces stamina. However, it is also used for ailments such as heartburn, indigestion, asthma, and high blood pressure. Additionally, Gondolosi has tested positive for vitamins A, D, E, and K and nutrients such as zinc, iron, magnesium, and calcium (Face of Malawi, 2017). The same is the case with Kigelia pinnata also known as Mvunguti; the fruit of the Mvunguti tree is traditionally used to enlarge muscles in both males and females. According to Dhungana et al. (2016), the Mvunguti tree has been used for generations in Africa to treat various ailments, such as malaria and diabetes. In addition, this fruit has therapeutic properties as it contains alkaloids and sterols. The Moringa tree, known for its pharmacological compounds, has recently been used in modern cosmetics in the production of skincare products, and it is also prescribed by practitioners of modern medicine (the synthesised version). According to Sagona et al. (2020), the leaves of the Moringa tree contain up to 25% of protein – hence its ability to improve muscle growth – and also boosts up to 90 nutrients and 46 antioxidants, including iron, zinc, and calcium.

6.5 WADA's Criteria vis-à-vis African Indigenous Remedies

WADA's efforts in controlling doping rely on the monitoring programmes instituted in all member countries. The monitoring institutions are entrusted with monitoring the development of medicines, reporting the effects of the medication, and providing information on the use of the drugs (WADA, 2021). However, the use of indigenous remedies in Africa is prevalent and, as this chapter argues, should be considered by WADA because it is dangerous to disregard traditional remedies and to violate WADA's criteria.

African people use traditional remedies because they believe they are safe. After all, Africans have been using them before Western medicine, and these remedies are part of their cultural and traditional heritage. However, many scientific researchers have argued that many of the plants/raw materials used in preparing these traditional remedies are potentially toxic. According to Fennell et al. (2004), the validation of plant use in the preparation of traditional remedies resulted from the presence of active compounds found in the plants. In addition, many of the plants used by practitioners of traditional medicine in Africa have the potential to cause cancer and cause gene mutations over time (Fennell et al., 2004). Thus, traditional remedies should be closely monitored because the materials used in preparing these remedies are potentially harmful and should be left in the hands of people who are knowledgeable on the matter. Further, the use of these remedies violates the WADA criterion, which states that a substance or method ought to be considered doping if it has the potential to harm or compromise an athlete's health.

The presence of active compounds in traditional remedies notwithstanding, these remedies can also be potentially harmful to an athlete's health because of the methods of preparation, methods of storage, as well as the amounts in which the treatments are prescribed. Additionally, the use of traditional medicine is not actively regulated in most African countries, which poses a threat to the health of athletes and the general population (Tamokou et al., 2014). The ability of the active compounds found in plants to alter genetic dispositions also goes against WADA's stipulation in the code. This is the case because gene mutation can be a source of inequality and goes against the spirit/integrity of sport, particularly the principle of a level playing field. WADA and other sports governing bodies have displayed inconsistencies in dealing with issues of genetic dispositions. For instance, Micheal Phelps has a genetic disposition that allows him to produce less lactic acid which gives him an advantage over other athletes (Lopez, 2021). Instead of dealing with this issue in the same way that world athletics have handled Semenya's case, Phelps is applauded for his condition. Additionally, when male athletes are found to have naturally high testosterone levels (above the average), they are allowed to compete, which is not the case for female athletes (Lopez, 2021) .

Even though some might argue that the effectiveness of traditional remedies rests on people's beliefs and not particularly on the fact that they have evidence to support effectiveness, it is part of performance enhancement for many African athletes. Traditional remedies are also contrary to WADA's stipulations because most of the materials used in the preparation are unknown to the athlete; in most cases, they are given concoctions made from different substances. WADA should also consider that because most athletes and traditional medicine practitioners do not know the composition of these traditional remedies, they become subject to unintentional doping, which, however, does not exempt them from punishment if they test positive for any of the substances on the prohibition list.

6.6 Conclusion

As this chapter has demonstrated, some traditional remedies violate the anti-doping criteria as prescribed by WADA and should therefore be considered for the prohibited list. Traditional remedies employed by African athletes as performance-enhancing agents clearly disregard the criteria outlined by WADA. It is commendable that some African sports governing bodies should have acted in cases where traditional remedies were employed for performance enhancement, as in the case of the Football Association of Malawi. To this effect, WADA should recognise that African indigenous traditional remedies are an integral part of the people's culture, and as such the issue of investigating and the possible inclusion of traditional remedies on WADA's watch list should be handled with utmost sensitivity. In recognition of the importance of traditional remedies to African people, the World Health Organization has made strides to ensure that public health policies consider traditional medicines by making sure that there are avenues where scientific evidence on the efficacy, quality, and safety of the remedies can be provided. The use of traditional remedies raises a variety of problems especially with regard to people's health.

A large part of the African population up to date still relies on the use of traditional remedies as part of their culture and tradition. Thus, it should not come as a surprise that African athletes employ traditional remedies in sports in a bid to improve their performance. It is against this background that this chapter urges WADA to formulate policies that can be employed for regulating the use of traditional remedies in sports. WADA should ensure that the monitoring programmes that are instituted in member countries pay attention to the development of these traditional remedies in a bid to uphold the principles that are stipulated in the anti-doping code. Zhang (2012) argues that it is important for governments of African countries to regulate the production and use of traditional remedies because they are associated with different health problems. At present, the use of modern analytical and pharmaceutical technologies makes it possible for standard herbal products to be made from standard herbal extracts. This makes it easy for organisations such as WADA to develop screening methods where it would be possible to test athletes for substances that are found in traditional remedies.

Future studies should focus on how WADA and other sports governing bodies can develop methodologies that can be used in ascertaining whether or not traditional remedies enhance sports performance. It is left to say that WADA should endeavour to roll out more programmes where athletes are provided with information on the preservation of the spirit of sport, level playing field, and protect their health and well-being. It is also important that WADA builds a better working relationship with athletes and not the current relationship where athletes are treated as irresponsible individuals. There is a need for WADA to make provisions for avenues where traditional remedies can be tested, thus providing scientific evidence on the efficacy of traditional remedies used in African sports. By including traditional remedies on the prohibition list, WADA would revamp the efforts that have been made in the war on doping in sports in addition to playing a pivotal role in the protection of the health of the general population in Africa because such efforts would be incorporated into public policy.

References

Bleak, J. L., and Frederick, C. M. (1998). Superstitious behavior in sport: levels of effectiveness and determinants of use in three collegiate sports. *Journal of Sport Behavior, 21*(1), 1–1.

Cocks, M., and Møller, V. (2002). Use of indigenous and indigenised medicines to enhance personal well-being: a South African case study. *Social Science and Medicine, 54*(3), 387–397.

Dhungana, B. J., Jyothi, Y., and Das, K. (2016). Kigelia Pinnata: exploration of potential medicinal usage in human ailments. *Journal of Pharmaceutical Research, 15*(4), 138–146.

Epstein, D. (2013). *The Sports Gene: Inside the Science of Extraordinary Athletic Performance*. Current.

Face of Malawi (September 19, 2017). Gondolosi Habours Health Benefits. Retrieved from www.faceofmalawi.com

Fennell, C. W., Lindsey, K. L., McGaw, L. J., Stafford, G. I., Elgorashi, G., and Van Staden, J. (2004). Assessing African medicinal plants for efficacy and safety: pharmacological screening and toxicology. *Ethnopharmacol, 94*(2–3), 205–217.

Geeraets, V. (2018). Ideology, doping and the spirit of sport". *Sports, Ethics and Philosophy, 12*(3), 255–271.

Gino, F., and Norton, M. (May 14, 2013). Why Rituals Work: There Are Real Benefits to Rituals, Religious or Otherwise. *Scientific American*. Available at www.scientificamerican.com/article/why-rituals-work/

Imray, G. (May 24, 2022). Semenya Says She Offered to Show Track Officials Her Body. *The Globe and Mail*. Available atwww.theglobeandmail.com/sports/olympics/article-semenya-says-she-offered-to-show-track-officials-her-body/

Kayser, B., and Smith, A. C. (2008). Globalisation of anti-doping: the reverse side of the medal. *BMJ (Clinical Research Ed.), 337*(7661), a584. https://doi.org/10.1136/bmj.a584

Kayser, B. A., and Mauron, M. A. (2007). Current anti-doping policy: a critical appraisal. *BMC Medical Ethics, 8*(2), 1–10 https://doi.org/10.1186/1472-6939-8-2

Kicman, A., and Gover, D. B. (2003). Anabolic steroids in sport: biochemical, clinical and analytical perspectives. *Annals of Clinical Biochemistry, 40*, 321–358.

Lopez, Q. (July 26, 2021). 4 top athletes barred from competing in either olympic events because their natural testosterone levels are deemed too high. *Business Insider*. Available at www.insider.com/intersex-olympic-athletes-barred-from-competing-in-preferred-olympic-event-2021-7

MacAuley, D. (1996). Drugs in sports. *British Medical Journal, 313*(7051), 211–215.

McGrath, M. (February 23, 2010). World Cup Players Face Herbal Medicine Tests. *Independent*. Available at www.independent.co.uk/sport/football/news/world-cup-players-face-herbal-medicine-tests-1907424.html

Morris, B. (1989). Medicine and herbalism in Malawi. *The Society of Malawi Journal, 42*(2), 34–54.

Muga, E. (2004). *Bewitching the Pitch in Tanzania*. BBC News Online.

Mulungwa, C., Holtzhansen, L. J., Joubert, G., and Mofolo, N. (2018). Exploring the use of African traditional medicines and rituals in South African professional football. *African Journal of Indigenous Knowledge Systems, 17*(2), 219–233.

Ndovi, J. (May 31, 2017). *4 Teams Fined for Juju Rituals*. The Nation Newspaper. Available at mwnation.com/4-teams-fined-for-juju-rituals/#:~:text=Four%20top%20Super%20League%20clubs,during%20Airtel%20Top%208%20matches.

Ngubane, H. (1977). *Body and Mind in Zulu Medicine: An Ethnography of Health and Disease in Nyuswa-Zulu Thought and Practice*. Academic Press, *31*, 22–27.

Nolte, K., Steyn, B. J. M., Kruger, P. E., and Flecher, L. (2014). Doping in sport: attitudes, beliefs and knowledge of competitive high-school athletes in Gauteng Province. *South African Journal of Sports Medicine*, *26*(3), 81–86.

Richter, M. (2003). *Traditional Medicines and Traditional Healers in South Africa*. Academia.

Sagona, W. C. J., Chirwa, P. W., and Sajidu, S. M. (2020). The miracle mix of Molinga: status of Molinga research and development in Malawi. *South African Journal of Botany*, *129*, 138–145.

Scientific American (May 1, 2019). "Natutally Occuring High Testosterone Shouldn't Keep Female Athletes Out of Competition." (2019, May 1). Retrieved from www.scientificamerican.com/article/naturally-occurring-high-testosterone-shouldn-t-keep-female-athletes-out-of-competition/#:~:text=There%20is%20no%20scientific%20basis,were%20revealed%20this%20past%20spring).

Smith, A., and Stewart, B. (2015). Why the war on drugs in sport will never be won. *Harm Reduction Journal*, *12*(53), 1–6.

Sofowora, A. (1996). Research on medicinal plants and traditional medicine in Africa. *Journal of Alternative and Contemplary Medicine*, *2*(3), 365–372.

Tamokou, J. D., and Kuete, V. (2014). "Toxic plants used in African traditional medicine". In V. Kuete (Ed.) *Toxicological Survey of African Medicinal Plants*. London: Elsevier. (pp. 135–180).

Vlad, R. A., Hancu, G., Popescu, G. C., and Lungu, L. A. (2018). Doping in sports, a never-ending story? *Advanced Pharmaceutical Bulletin*, *8*(4), 529–534.

World Anti-Doping Agency (2021). *World Anti-Doping Code*. Montreal (Canada): World Anti-Doping Agency. Available at www.wada-ama.org/en/what-we-do/world-anti-doping-code

Yuan, H., Ma, Q., Ye, L., and Piao, G. (2016). The traditional medicine and modern medicine from natural products. *Molecule*, *21*(5), 559.

Zhang, J., Wider, B., Shang, H., Li, X., and Ernst, E. (2012). Quality of herbal medicines: challenges and solutions. *Complementary Therapies in Medicine*. *20*(1–2), 100–106.

Chapter 7

Socio-Economic Context and Doping in Africa

Jean-Christophe Lapouble

7.1 Introduction

The fight against doping in Africa cannot be approached without placing this fight in the more global context of African countries, for which the issue of doping is only an epiphenomenon amid all the challenges these countries must face. Nor can the fight against doping be considered a priority within public policy, given socio-economic factors. Even if the indices relating to economic development or human development can be criticised, it seems interesting to us to situate the African continent with some indicators to be able to describe the actual situation of the fight against doping and not a situation based solely on the ratification by most African countries of the World Anti-Doping Code as required by the 2005 United Nations Educational, Scientific and Cultural Organization (UNESCO, 2005) Global Convention on Doping, which was adopted at the global level by 191 countries, including almost all African countries except Guinea-Bissau and South Sudan.

It appears that the fight against doping in Africa cannot be considered in a theoretical manner, that is, taken out of its socio-economic context. The experience of the Coronavirus disease 2019 (Covid-19) epidemic in Africa has clearly shown that the response modalities of African countries cannot be the same as those of other countries. Indeed, the organisation of the public health system and the public administration, in general, contributed to the effectiveness of the response. Therefore, there is no reason to believe that the fight against doping, as much a matter of education as public health, is not influenced by such elements. So, we will look at the level of development freedom of association, the state of the administration in general, corruption, and public health. These elements are not without consequences in the fight against doping in African countries.

7.2 Economic Development

To understand better the framework in which anti-doping policies in Africa should be applied, we thought of looking at a few indicators such as gross

DOI: 10.4324/9781003370796-8

domestic product (GDP) per capita, the poverty rate, the peace index, and the human development index. These different indicators, imperfect as they may be, nevertheless allow us to understand that the fight against doping in Africa cannot be a priority but a policy carried out in a residual manner in certain states that have a particular interest in doing so, such as winning medals at the Olympic Games, because the registration of athletes can only be carried out insofar as the latter undertake to respect the World Anti-Doping Code.

It is very clear that the GDP per capita in Africa is the lowest of the five continents over the period from 1970 to 2019 even if this data conceals significant differences between countries (Acemoglu, 2003). Thus, the average in Africa is US$1,884 for 2019, while for the most favoured continent in North America it is US$42,796. The GDP in Africa varies from US$17,052 for the Seychelles to US$275 in South Sudan. The latter country has recorded a 78% drop compared to the previous period. It thus appears that in Africa significant drops in GDP are not uncommon, which is certainly a peculiarity of this continent.

In 2019, countries with the highest poverty rate at the US$2.15-a-day poverty line were mostly in Sub-Saharan Africa (Word Bank, 2022, p. 37). Poverty remains highly concentrated in Sub-Saharan Africa, with a poverty rate that is about four times higher than that of the second poorest region in the world, and the evidence on the pace of poverty reduction in the region is unaffected (World Bank, 2023, p. 38). If we address the question of the human development index (United Nations Development Programme, 2021/2022, p. 311), among the 66 countries that are listed as having a very high level of human development, there are no African countries. The highest index is obtained by Switzerland (0.962). The first African country is Algeria which is in 91st place (index 0.745). South Sudan is in 191st and last place with an index of 0.385 for 2021.

According to the Global Peace Index (GPI) analysis,

> Sub-Saharan Africa recorded a slight fall in peacefulness in the 2022 GPI, with the average country score deteriorating by 0.022 points, or one per cent. Of the 44 countries in the region, 21 improved in score, while 22 deteriorated and one remained unchanged.
>
> (Institute for Economics and Peace 2022, p. 21)

When reading these different indicators, it is clear that the fight against doping cannot be a major issue in Africa as there are other urgent matters to be dealt with. It is appropriate to ask whether such a fight is not an unattainable luxury whose social utility is questionable.

7.3 Associations

In the sports world, most clubs and federations are set up as non-profit associations. This legal form, which may seem harmless, does not appear to be a legal structure whose creation is free in many countries, where the risk of creating an opposition political party leads to controls and provisions that sometimes make the creation of associations very difficult. Article 20 of the Universal Declaration of Human Rights provides that everyone has the right to freedom of peaceful assembly and association and that no one may be compelled to belong to an association. The Banjul Charter (1981) guarantees in its article 10 the freedom of association in the following form:

> 1. Every individual shall have the right to free association provided that he abides by law. 2. Subject to the obligation of solidarity provided for in 29 no one may be compelled to join an association.

Article 29 of this Charter provides for a number of duties to be respected, including the obligation not to jeopardise the security of the state.

Moreover, freedom of association also includes the freedom to form a trade union. This freedom is also guaranteed by international conventions adopted under the aegis of the International Labour Organization (ILO), especially number 50 and number 51. Thus, freedom of association is a strong marker of democratic development in general, but also of the reality of collective bargaining: "the exercise of freedom of association and the right to collective bargaining are based on the defence of fundamental civil liberties, including the right to liberty and security of person, freedom of opinion, expression and assembly, the right to a fair trial by an impartial and independent tribunal, and the right to protection of property of employers' organisations and trade unions" (Bureau International du Travail, 2008, p. 5). ILO Convention 87 concerns freedom of association and protection of the right to organise. Convention No. 98 concerns the application of the principles of the right to organise and collective bargaining. As for the Banjul Charter, a large majority of African countries have ratified these two conventions (over 90%) since 1950.

What can be observed in both common law and civil law countries is that, in general, sports associations do not seem to have any particular difficulty in being legally constituted, even in countries where the freedom of association is closely controlled. Indeed, the declared (if not proven) apolitical nature of the sports world in general and of the International Olympic Committee in particular does not lead states to exercise close control over the creation and functioning of sports clubs (Lapouble, 2011). The list of National Olympic Committees recognised by the International Olympic Committee (IOC, 2023) shows that the creation of a structure of this type is not particularly difficult.

7.4 Public Administration

The state of the administration in Africa can be understood with some international indicators. It should be noted, however, that the indicators never refer to the administrations in charge of sport. It is true that, depending on the country, if this type of administration exists, it may be attached to the education or health sector. Even if the Doing Business index is no longer published until another index is, data on the quality of the administration in each country can be mentioned, at least to give an overall state of the administration. Given that sports administration is rarely on the government's agenda, the indications given at the aggregate level can help to assess the state of sports administration in various African countries. Overall, it is clear that some regions of the world are more favourable for doing business and it is clear that many African countries are poorly ranked (Doing Business, 2020, p. 32).

As a first step, it may be interesting to look at the overall score for the different indicators included in the Doing Business ranking, which gives an idea of the modernisation and efficiency of the administration of the countries in question. For example, it is possible to analyse the data for Sub-Saharan Africa (Doing Business, 2020, p. 5). Overall, few African countries are ranked in the top 100 (for the global indicator) although the first is Mauritius, ranked 13th with an index of 81.5, while most other Sub-Saharan African countries are ranked after the top 100. The last country ranked with an index of 20 is Somalia (ranked 190). In terms of sectoral indicators, on a maximum base of 100, the best score achieved is 80.1 for starting a business, but other indicators can be much lower (Resolving Insolvency: 31.3).

If we take two indicators among others, such as the connection to electricity and the payment of taxes, this can give an idea of the state of the administration in general, which is certainly imperfect, but insofar as the administration in charge of sport is not a priority, it is difficult to imagine that the two indicators chosen do not constitute priorities for African countries, since they are markers in terms of development. In other words, if these indicators are not good, there is no reason to believe that the administration of sport in the country (with extraordinary exceptions) can be in a satisfactory state.

Thus, it appears that the time to obtain an electricity connection in the area concerned is longer than it is in the rest of the world. Moreover, this average reflects huge disparities between countries such as Liberia where the connection time was 482 days in 2020 compared to 37 days in Rwanda.

In terms of the number of payments to be made, the cumbersome nature of most African administrations is evident. Tanzania's index is 59, while South Africa's index is 7 for a regional average of 36.6. It is also possible to take a more basic indicator of the functioning of administrations essential to the population, such as the registration of births, which also concerns the entire population and not primarily the urban population. There was an increase of 2% in the proportion of under-five children whose births were registered in Africa from 49% in 2008 to 51% in 2020. Projection scenarios built on existing trend show that, unless progress is accelerated, the number of unregistered children in Africa will continue to rise and will exceed 100 million by 2030 (World Health Organization, 2022, p. 114). These elements, which globally show a poor functioning of the administration in general, can lead one to think that the administrations in charge of the fight against doping are not very structured, nor very efficient. Information from WADA corroborates this observation.

The provisions of the World Anti-Doping Code state that in each country an independent agency should be responsible for the fight against doping (Lapouble, 2001). Article 20.5 and following of the World Anti-Doping Code (Miège and Lapouble, 2004; WADA, 2021) govern the conditions for the implementation of such an agency. Thus, the agency must be independent and free of any conflict of interest with respect to both sports organisations and the government. In terms of education, this is the responsibility of national anti-doping agencies (WADA, 2023). In terms of funding, even though Africa's contribution has been limited to 0.5% of the total budget, which represents US$46 million in 2023, each African country must contribute an amount that varies from US$802 for countries such as Malawi or Somalia to US$5,141 for South Africa (WADA, 2023). The total amount of these contributions is certainly modest ($117,924), but given the lack of resources, it is difficult to see how such a small amount can help WADA's operations, even though, due to an under-resourced administration, anti-doping programmes are almost non-existent. It is true that a distinction must be made between the contribution due and the contribution actually paid. Thus, for the year 2022 (WADA, 2022), only $59,541 was actually collected by WADA for a total amount of $109,189. It should be noted that South Africa is in a special situation in the fight against doping because not only does it have the only analytical laboratory on the African continent but also a local WADA office in the city of Cape Town.

However, it is important to qualify this observation, which suggests that anti-doping tests are not carried out. Indeed, the analysis of the controls carried out in Athletics in Africa allows to have a more nuanced vision. Obviously, athletics is the sport that brings the most medals to African countries.

The data provided by WADA for the year 2021 (WADA 2021) shows that Kenya is ranked 8th in the world in terms of controls in this discipline (684 controls), just before Spain, which indicates that at the level of controls some African anti-doping organisations are doing real work (Lapouble, 2017). The other African countries that follow in the ranking are Morocco, South Africa, and Nigeria, respectively. However, at the global level, only 19 African countries have carried out controls in athletics. Some, like Burkina Faso, have done only one. The same applies to Ivory Coast. Given the political and economic situation of Burkina Faso, this figure is not surprising. On the other hand, it is much more surprising for Ivory Coast, whose indicators in terms of administrative efficiency are much better. This shows that if the global state of the administration of a state can be correlated with the state of the administration in charge of sport, there are always particularities. Thus, Egypt has carried out 162 controls, which is the 5th rank among African countries, while this country is ranked 114 in Doing Business. However, the number of audits carried out in Egypt is just higher than those carried out in Norway, ranked 7 in Doing Business. However, these differences can be well explained. The population of the two countries is not at all comparable (110 million in Egypt versus 5.5 million in Norway). In addition, athletics is not a sport that is widely practised in Norway.

Another indicator of the weakness of controls is the number of analyses carried out by the South African laboratory, the only one accredited in Africa, which carried out a little less than 1.65% of the world total in 2021 (WADA 2021). It should be noted that not all samples taken in Africa are necessarily analysed there. At the level of the anti-doping administrations themselves, one can only note that the obligation of independence from the sports movement as requested by WADA is not always respected. This is particularly the case when tests are conducted by a national Olympic Committee, as in Botswana, Rwanda, Tanzania, Namibia, or Madagascar. It is true that the principle of independence is not respected either when the test is requested by the Ministry of Sports, as in Lesotho.

Faced with these shortcomings, the aid proposed by the Olympic movement to structure African sport does not seem sufficient. The Olympic Solidarity Program does not provide for specific aid for the establishment of national anti-doping agencies. Even though Africa is the leading continent in terms of Olympic Solidarity (Olympic Solidarity and NOC Services, 2021), with 54 National Olympic Committees, there is no budget line that directly concerns the fight against doping and the support of national anti-doping agencies. In fact, the aid mainly concerns aid for teams so that they can participate in the Olympic Games or individual grants for athletes. However, there is a specific programme designed to help structure national Olympic committees or local sports federations, such as the one in Cape Verde (Olympic Solidarity and NOC Services, 2021, p. 7). In terms of initiatives carried out specifically in Africa, it appears that the fight against doping is addressed through workshops or, in some cases, the payment of the contribution due by some countries to WADA (Olympic Solidarity and NOC Services, 2021, p. 30). There is a specific programme aimed at structuring National Olympic Committees but that is not specific to the fight against doping (Olympic Solidarity and NOC Services, 2021, p. 29) to ensure the implementation of good governance practices. The amount of this programme at the global level for the year 2021 amounts to $18,875,000. Within this framework, 50 African Olympic Committees have been assisted (Olympic Solidarity and NOC Services, 2021, p. 53). To promote the values of Olympism, the Olympafrica Foundation helps support community centres. (Olympic Solidarity and NOC Services, 2021, p. 36).

7.5 Corruption

According to Alina Mungiu-Pippidi (2015, p. 116), "Corruption emerges when someone has monopoly power over a good or service, has the discretion to decide who receives it and how much they receive, and is not accountable". However, it is clear that the sports world is essentially based on a series of monopolies entrusted to non-governmental organisations with little control (Graycan and Russel-Smith, 2011).

Sport is not immune to corruption and it must be recognised that if the level of corruption in a country is high, there is no reason to think that the sports world will be spared. Thus, even in countries where corruption is the lowest, corruption cases can reach the sports movement (Sport, Transparency International, 2016). In the field of doping, there is no reason to think that corruption does not affect the sports world, especially since some cases have led to the exclusion of Russia from international competitions because of manipulations during the analysis of the Sochi Olympic Games. The Court of Arbitration for Sports recognised the non-conformity of the actions of the Russian Anti-Doping Agency in a decision of 17 December 2020. These actions are not isolated and had given rise in the past to other errors, particularly in terms of access to data from the Anti-Doping Administration and Management System (ADAMS) (Cyling news, 2016). Cases relating to corruption in the fight against doping have thus affected African countries, such as Kenya in 2015 (Clarey, 2015) or Senegal with the former president of the International Federation of Athletics in 2016 who was convicted by the French justice for corruption (Bouchez, 2020).

Overall, Africa's corruption ranking is clearly not satisfactory (Transparency International, 2021). Sub-Saharan Africa has the worst score, with an average score of 33, the lowest among all regions in the world. This score reflects a wide range of situations, none of which is satisfactory. The worst score is for South Sudan (11/100), while the Seychelles has the best score (70/100) (Transparency International, 2021, p. 14). We can notice that the two other countries that stand out are Cape Verde (58/100) and Botswana (55/100). If we look at the Middle East and North Africa zone, the global score is hardly better as it is 39, just after Eastern Europe and Asia.

The findings on the level of sports organisations are not very encouraging. According to Transparency International (2016), Africa remains stunted by a combination of talent drain (mainly to Europe), a lack of government investment and policy guidelines, corruption, and gross mismanagement. The report adds that major events are a main avenue of abuse and corruption in sport in Africa. Faced with such an observation, it is not surprising that efforts are being made to improve the functioning of African sports organisations, even if it seems illusory to want to make sports organisations function in a transparent manner in an environment that is not transparent.

Within the framework of the Olympic Solidarity Program, some actions are carried out in the field of integrity education as well as to promote the good governance of sports organisations (Olympic Solidarity and NOC Services, p. 43). It is certainly no coincidence that the assistance given to the structuring of the Olympic Committee has been successful, given the low level of corruption in this country (Olympic Solidarity and NOC Services, p. 30). These elements are corroborated by the analysis of the number of controls carried out by Cape Verde in Athletics (18 controls) for a population of 562,000 inhabitants (WADA, 2021, p. 47). It is thus clear that the fight against corruption in Africa in the field of anti-doping must take on a transnational dimension (Hatchard, 2014, p. 333).

7.6 Public Heath

Insofar as the fight against doping is often presented as a public health problem, it must be noted that in the face of the health challenges facing the African continent, the issue of the fight against doping appears to be a marginal phenomenon. In fact, since the Covid-19 epidemic has severely tested all the health systems in the world, it is clear that African countries have only been able to face such a challenge with limited means. Therefore, the African continent has a population that represents 14.4% of the world population, but accounts for only 1% of the global health spending (World Health Organization, 2022). As the maps show, access to basic health services is still not guaranteed for a large part of the African population.

As the fight against doping is also a fairly sophisticated medical field, it is easy to understand that most African countries are not in a position to implement prevention and/or repression policies. The level of health emergency on the continent shows that doping prevention can only be a very specific policy, especially when Olympic medals are at stake. Moreover, the effective implementation of Athlete Biological Passport is a challenge for African athletes.

Currently only one anti-doping laboratory is accredited for the entire African continent, namely, the South African Doping Control Laboratory in Bloemfontein (WADA, 2023). Faced with a lack of equipment and limited road infrastructure, Africa may be an interesting fallback for some non-African athletes to carry outdoping product cures such as anabolic agents whose effects persist over time, even though detection must be carried out within a limited period of time after taking them. Having made this assumption at the time of the generalisation of out-of-competition testing with the implementation of the ADAMS system, it appears that some athletes have tried to take advantage of the difficulties of access to Africa to avoid testing. For example, a French athlete went to train in Marrakech where she failed to be tested, resulting in a four-year ban from competitions by Conseil d'Etat, the French higher administrative court.

7.7 Conclusion

At the end of this analysis, it is very clear that the ratification by almost all African countries of the UNESCO Convention on doping and therefore the adoption of the World Anti-Doping Code is, for many countries, a mere display measure, as much more important priorities remain to be addressed. Rather than asking the countries which are *de jure* forced to ratify a convention that they know they cannot apply in order for their athletes to participate in international competitions, we should question the blatant shortcomings of WADA , which imposes legislation that it knows will not be applied. It is a pity that we prefer the display to the recognition of the enormous difficulties encountered in the field. As far as the fight against doping in Africa is concerned, one can only regret this inflation of normative texts, which are inapplicable considering the problems that this continent is facing. In other words, in view of the African socio-economic context, the application of the World Anti-Doping Code constitutes a legislative doping without real effect in most of the states.

References

Acemoglu, D. (2003). An African success story: Bostwana. In D. Rodrick (Ed.), *In Search of Prosperity: Analytic Narrative on Economic Growth*. Princeton: Princeton University Press.

Bouchez, Y. (2020, September 16). *Corruption au sein de la fédération internationale d'athlétisme: les six prévenus, dont son ex-patron Lamine Diack, condamnés*. Available at www.lemonde.fr/sport/article/2020/09/16/corruption-au-sein-de-la-federation-internationale-d-athletisme-les-six-prevenus-condamnes_6052486_3242.html

Bureau International du Travail. (2008, 28-mai–13 juin). *Conférence internationale du travail, 97e session*. Available at www.ilo.org/ilc/ILCSessions/previous-sessions/97thSession/lang--fr/index.htm

Clarey, C. (2015, November 30). Cloud of corruption and doping hangs worldwide. *New York Times*. Available at www.nytimes.com/2015/12/01/sports/kenyan-track-doping-suspension-iaaf-hamburg-olympics.html?searchResultPosition=1

Cycling News. (2016, October 6). WADA details response to Fancy Bears' hacking. https://www.cyclingnews.com/news/wada-details-response-to-fancy-bears-hacking/

Graycar, A., & Russel-Smith, G. (Eds.) (2011). *Handbook of Global Research and Practice in Corruption*. Cheltenham: Edward Elgar.

Hatchard, J. (2014). *Combating Corruption: Legal Approaches to Supporting Good Governance and Integrity in Africa*. Cheltenham: Edward Elgar Publishing.

Institute for Economics and Peace (2022), *Global Peace Index 2022: Measuring peace in A complex world*. Sydney: Institute for Economics & Peace. Available at www.visionofhumanity.org/wp-content/uploads/2022/06/GPI-2022-web.pdf

IOC. (2023). National Olympic Committees. International Olympic Committee. Retrieved at https://olympics.com/ioc/national-olympic-committees

Lapouble, J. C. (2001). L'intervention publique en matière de dopage. *Revue française d'administration publique, 97,* 117–129.

Lapouble, J. C. (2011). La localisation des sportifs: une atteinte excessive à la vie privée ou quand Big Brother s'invite chez les sportifs. *Revue Trimestrielle des droits de l'Homme, 88,* 913–939.

Lapouble, J. C. (2017). Athletes whereabout in the context of the fight against doping in Africa; Mission; Impossible? *African Sport Law and Business Bulletin, 1,* 1–8.

Miège, C. and Lapouble, J. C. (2004). Sport et organisations internationales. *Economica Paris,* 215–227.

Mungiu-Pippidi, C. (2015). *The Quest for Good Governance: How Societies Develop Control of Corruption*. Cambridge: Cambridge University Press.

Olympic Solidarity and NOC Services. (2021). Annual report. Available at https://indd.adobe.com/view/ed907367-7288-4986-adfd-f0b2a222dd26

Organization of African Unity (1981). *The Banjul Charter*. Available at https://au.int/sites/default/files/treaties/36390-treaty-0011_-_african_charter_on_human_and_peoples_rights_f.pdf

Transparency International. (2016). *Global Corruption Report: Sport*. London and New York: Routledge. Available at https://baselgovernance.org/sites/default/files/2019-02/2016_gcrsport_en.pdf

Transparency International. (2021). *Indices de perception de la corruption*. Available at https://transparency-france.org/publications/indices-de-perception-de-corruption/

UNESCO. (2005). *International Convention against Doping in Sport*. Available at https://unesdoc.unesco.org/ark:/48223/pf0000142594

United Nations Development Programme. (2021/2022). *Uncertain Times; Unsettled Lives: Shaping our Future in a Transforming World.*

WADA. (2021). *World Anti-Doping Code 2021*. Available at www.wada-ama.org/sites/default/files/resources/files/2021_wada_code.pdf.

WADA. (2022). *Anti-Doping Testing Figures*. Available at www.wada-ama.org/en/resources/anti-doping-stats/anti-doping-testing-figures-report

WADA. (2023). Contributions au Budget de l'Ama Pour 2022. Available at www.wada-ama.org/sites/default/files/2023-01/wada_contributions_2022_update_fr.pdf

World Bank. (2020). *Doing Business: region profile: Sub-Saharan Africa*. Available at www.doingbusiness.org/content/dam/doingBusiness/media/Profiles/Regional/DB2020/SSA.pdf

World Bank. (2023). *Doing Business: Poverty and Shared Prosperity 2022: Correcting Course*. Available at https://openknowledge.worldbank.org/server/api/core/bitstreams/b96b361a-a806-5567-8e8a-b14392e11fa0/content

World Health Organization. (2022). *Atlas of African Health Statistics: health situation analysis of the WHO African Region — country profiles*. Available at https://apps.who.int/iris/handle/10665/364837.

Part II

African Practice and Doping

Chapter 8

Framing Anti-Doping Initiatives in Malawian Sports News

Mwaona Nyirongo

8.1 Introduction

Doping, or using forbidden performance-enhancing substances, is one of Malawi's most significant obstacles to athletic progress (Kaoche, 2019). Vipene (2003, p. 103) points out that doping has negative consequences such as memory loss, addiction, and hallucinations. Kaoche et al. (2020) observe that doping drives away sponsors, shatters relationships, and destroys innate talent in sports. Malawian news outlets have covered anti-doping stories, assisting in shaping anti-doping narratives. The amount of research on these news items is minimal, making it difficult for decision-makers to decide how to proceed with their anti-doping campaign, especially in mediated spaces. This chapter investigates how anti-doping news is presented in Malawian sports news.

The World Anti-Doping Agency (WADA) determines whether an athlete is doping or not through laboratory examinations of blood and urine, which employ a variety of metrics for either screening or detecting the use of prohibited drugs and procedures. These lab tests are conducted at WADA-approved facilities that follow the International Organization for Standardization (ISO) 17025 standard because the results can be used to charge and potentially sanction athletes (Banfi et al., 2010, p. 1003). Anti-doping testing employs haematology, proteins, hormones, and isoelectric focusing (IEF). The haematological method focuses on blood testing in particular and measures like haemoglobin (Hb), haematocrit (Ht), and reticulocyte count (Ret). The proteins technique focuses on indirect markers for detecting recombinant human erythropoietin (rHuEpo) abuse and measuring soluble transferrin receptor (sTfR) (Banfi et al., 2010, p. 1004). Hormonal testing includes looking at recombinant growth hormone (rhGH), which is used as a doping agent due to its anabolic properties (it increases lean body mass and decreases fat, enhancing power). Although it has not been proven definitively that rhGH improves athletic performance, it is widely used in certain sports, particularly when combined with steroids (Banfi et al., 2010, p. 1006). Finally, IEF tests detect Epo and related compounds (biosimilars) in urine. Banfi et al. (2010, p. 1005) aver that the recombinant form

DOI: 10.4324/9781003370796-10

of Epo (HuEpo) was initially developed to treat anaemia. However, athletes immediately misappropriated it to stimulate erythropoiesis and, as a result, oxygen availability in peripheral tissues such as muscles.

Banfi et al. (2010, p. 1007) have urged the scientific community to stop lying to the world about how trustworthy, safe, and effective anti-doping techniques are in ensuring doping-free competitions. The techniques are not as safe, realistic, or effective as scientists promise; they do not encourage anti-doping sports. Banfi et al. (2010) further propose that:

> Laboratory medicine professionals and their scientific associations can support the ongoing effort of anti-doping laboratories in fighting cheats through the evidence of proper methodology, correct and effective inter-methods comparison, the experience of external quality control and proficiency testing. The collaborative studies involving anti-doping and laboratory medicine experts will stimulate the diffusion within the scientific community of the enormous quantity of data collected on "clean" athletes, representing an incomparable background for evaluating physiology and improving knowledge in sports medicine.
>
> (p. 1007)

Anti-doping tests have come under criticism from the laboratory medicine community and the general public. Møller (2014) addresses severe concerns voiced by athletes concerning the efficiency of and commitment to anti-doping. In November 2011, for example, over 100 player unions representing over 150,000 working athletes convened to discuss issues affecting their careers. During the meeting, representatives discussed the Anti-Doping Code, stating that they support solid anti-doping regulations but disagree with the WADA Code. They published a very critical evaluation of WADA where the athletes stated that they were not adequately involved in developing the code; hence, it was not representative of their will.

Møller (2014) reveals that the participants questioned WADA's legal underpinning as follows:

> It is inconsistent with fighting for fairness in sports using means that contravene civilised society's basic "rules" (human rights). [...] For working athletes, anti-doping rules and the resulting sanctions treat anti-doping rule violations as criminal. Working athletes will lose their livelihood if they do not consent to anti-doping rules; therefore, the consent is "nonvoluntary". Likewise, the consequence for working athletes of imposed sanctions and public shaming can be a loss of their livelihood. A system that denies them their procedural rights (i.e. under Article 6 EHCR) may not be imposed. The current system is legally unstable and subject to challenge on human rights grounds.
>
> (p. 935)

As evidenced by the committee members' statements above, athletes found to be doping are subjected to discipline and punishment. Writing on punishment and discipline, Foucault (1995) contends that punishment has changed in that it used to be physical but has become less physical as time has progressed. He adds that this evolution is not driven by a humanitarian desire but rather by a reaction to power systems that allow people to punish others more effectively and less cruelly. As a result, modern punishment focuses on the soul rather than the physical body for onlookers to feel the punishment, generate a visual representation that would deter others from committing a crime, and incentivise offenders to avoid devoting a crime rather than risk being punished.

Despite doping being associated with punishment and discipline, some athletes continue to dope to win, psychologically prepare for sports, improve their self-image, impress coaches, fulfil sponsor contractual obligations, and satisfy peer pressure (Kaoche et al., 2020, p. 6). Kaoche et al. (2020, p. 7) observed that hormones, stimulants, amino acids, and anabolic steroids were all identified as doping substances by football players and coaches in Malawi (88.9%, 82.1%, 80%, and 77%, respectively). According to the study, 77% of the athletes had a high level of anti-doping knowledge, 22.1% had a medium level of awareness, and 0.9% had a poor level of understanding. Friends, team doctors, and seminars provided the knowledge.

Although the athletes in Malawi acknowledged Western doping tactics among themselves, African players occasionally dope using African techniques that are discursively regarded as superstition in Western epistemology. Nyamnjoh (2019) notes that Africans believe in humanity's incompleteness, which leads them to seek ways to improve themselves through various methods, including magic, also known as *Juju*. He associates *Juju* with technology, but improving human capacities is also used in sports, with Africans, notably Malawians, attempting to use *Juju* to compensate for their weaknesses and thrive in sports. Arising from this understanding, it could be argued that *Juju* technology and innovation are also a form of doping. Njororai (2019, p. 99) states that *Juju* is so prevalent in Africa that the perception of who wins or loses a game is sometimes based on who has the finest witch doctor. Players in Africa are exposed to *Juju* from a young and sensitive age, making it tough to eliminate it from sports. Because it is not openly discussed, *Juju* is a well-hidden secret. When a team has identified the enemy team's *Juju*, they can develop an antidote to neutralise it (Njororai, 2019, p. 105). Even though *Juju* is prohibited in African football, it is far from being eradicated, as many of the sport's top managers also firmly believe in the occult.

Kovač (2016) perceives *Juju* as "spiritual doping", where actions in the spiritual world have immediate and significant effects on the material world. The stories of *Juju* are usually heard through rumours because of the secrecy surrounding *Juju* and accusations which revolve around the use of herbs, pieces of tree bark, or small thread which teams acquire from healers. The players are urged to drink, wash their hands, or put their feet in concoctions. These enhance performance and allow players to make miraculous moves. The West, and Fédération Internationale de Football Association (FIFA) in particular, are sceptical of the chemical composition of *Juju* while ignoring their more significant spiritual attributes. *Juju* is usually dismissed as a psychological delusion or superstition, but players constantly accuse each other for evidence of *Juju*. Sometimes *Juju* is used to injure opponent team members to win matches (Uroš, 2016).

Journalists play a crucial role in combating doping in sports by uncovering wrongdoing. Journalists have contributed information to WADA's anti-doping investigations (World Anti-Doping Agency, 2022). The media also informs the public about anti-doping activities around the world. Mwangi (2018, p. 15) claims that in 2015 WADA observed a growing relationship between the anti-doping community and sports journalists in promoting clean sports. In a study titled "Role of the Media in Curbing Doping among Middle and Long-Distance Runners in Kenya", Mwangi (2018, p. 39) found that 71.8% of the respondents agreed that the media helps in educating the masses, while only 17.8% disagreed with this fact. Furthermore, 56.2% believed that the media was a source of anti-doping information, while 31.4% disagreed.

The media's exposure of sports cheaters is critical because it deters players from taking activities that could jeopardise their lives if they are discovered. Journalists prefer to frame anti-doping in specific world views when reporting on doping. Mwangi (2018) further argues that the framing can be apparent in their vocabulary, such as using the term "cheating" rather than "doping" and referencing anti-doping advocates. Individual perceptions of persons in a group are emphasised in the media. As a result, the group works to make its favourite individuals popular with the general population, while those at odds with the authorities are humiliated. This understanding is helpful for general organisational tasks, although framing in sports isn't as elaborate.

Although journalists are critical in the fight, Mwangi (2018, p. 13) maintains that they lack adequate anti-doping training. Most of them learned about anti-doping from experience rather than thorough academic preparation, which leaves a significant gap in normative conceptualisation and reporting. Media lacks authoritative knowledge of anti-doping news, making it difficult for them to generate high-quality reporting, and public trust in our journalists is low. Furthermore, because doping has only lately gained traction in Africa, most media are still unfamiliar with the problem. Mwangi (2018, p. 41) elucidates that although media houses in Kenya host professional development seminars, they rarely host seminars on anti-doping reportage.

8.2 Theoretical Framework

This study engaged framing, agenda-setting, and dissonance theories from journalism and communication studies. Maxwell E. McCombs and Donald

L. Shaw created the agenda-setting theory after noticing that the media significantly affects the salience of issues and public leaders. McCombs, Shaw, and Weaver (2014) argue that the media influences public agenda regarding the salience of the attributes of these objects and the networked media agenda of objects or attributes on the networked public agenda of object or attribute prominence serves as a manifestation of the impact. Agenda-setting occurs on three levels, with the first assessing the story that must be reported on and the second examining how the general public should perceive the issue. This is where the sensationalism of news takes root to pique the audience's interest. The media also engages in priming, which is making a certain subject appear important by reporting on it regularly. The news is also presented in a specific frame of reference, which is later embraced by the general public. The WHAT and HOW of sports reporting are controlled by gatekeepers such as editors and news providers who influence the framing of news. This theory was essential in understanding how the news media framesets are engineered to influence how society understands anti-doping messages.

The framing theory of mass communication investigates how the media packages and presents information to the public. The theory builds on the agenda-setting theory by focusing on the issues being discussed rather than the topic itself. In this way, the media concentrates on specific occurrences to give them a particular meaning. According to the theory, how something is presented to people – the frame – impacts their decisions. The frames affect how the general public perceives news and, therefore, it may be thought of as a second level of agenda-setting theory in which they not only tell people what to think about (agenda setting) but also how to think about the issue (second-level agenda setting, framing theory) (Framing Theory, 2011). Goffman was the first to propose the idea, claiming that framing encompasses both natural and social realms. The natural function entails literally accepting the natural quote without referencing societal conceptions. The construct considers meaning as something that people create to achieve their objectives. Natural functions are frequently the source of social conceptions. Fairhurst and Sarr (1996) suggested the following tools for framing:

1 Metaphor: comparing something to something else to frame it.
2 Stories (myths, legends): a method of framing an event by associating it with a vividly remembered occurrence.
3 Tradition (rituals, ceremonies): using culturally relevant artefacts to tell stories.
4 Slogan, jargon, and catchphrase: using a memorable word to frame an event so that others could remember it.
5 Artefact: objects that hold more meaning than themselves.
6 Contrast: to explain something by describing what it isn't.
7 Spin: creating a bias of value judgement.

Framing theory is tied to agenda-setting theory because they both focus on how the media attracts the public attention. Framing theory investigates how the media consciously creates a frame for information (Framing Theory, 2011). The theory was critical in understanding how journalists choose news topics and reinforce the themes in those news items (Framing Theory, 2012).

To further understand how the news affects the mind, the study will also engage the cognitive dissonance theory, where cognitive dissonance is a mental clash or stress caused by acquiring knowledge or understanding through the senses, which eventually leads to a person changing his/her life choices. The cognitive dissonance theory helped in knowing how reporters use mental clashes or tension to persuade athletes to refrain from doping (Communication, 2012). This theory was proposed by Leon Festinger in the 1950s, indicating that people want to appear rational and consistent in their thoughts and actions. As a result, whenever one is confronted with the knowledge that contradicts this goal, they work hard to restore homeostasis so that the discomfort or inner discord might be reduced. People accomplish this by downplaying the dissonant thought's relevance, outweighing the discordant thought with a harmonious thought, or incorporating the discordant thought into their belief system.

This study aims to figure out how media frame anti-doping news and the kind of sport subject they project. The study also looks into how journalists try to persuade their audiences to change their habits to assist minimising drug use. The researcher will then evaluate how mind crush is applied to the frames to persuade the audience to adopt anti-doping messages. Allied research questions include the following: what are the anti-doping messages that journalists are trying to convey? What are the journalists' framing strategies for these messages? How do the journalists try to influence the masses using the messages? How do the messages create a crush of mind in the audience?

8.3 Research Design

This study took a qualitative research design referenced within the interpretative tradition (Bryman, 1988). Qualitative research was critical in gathering rich data based on subjective interpretations of texts and lived experiences (Creswell et al., 2007). A qualitative design was chosen to get an in-depth view of the anti-doping fight in the news reports; the researcher had no interest in replicating the findings unless it is carefully done by considering the environment in which one wants to replicate (Ntaba, 2012). The researcher conducted a qualitative content analysis of news reports from the *Times Group* and *Nation Online* from the year 2014 to 2021 to identify anti-doping messages, how they were framed and what the journalists wanted their audience to think about, how to think them through, and how to sustain such thoughts. At the same time, the content analysis probed how the reporters set the plan to influence the minds of their audience as far as the perception of the issue is concerned. And lastly, the analysis explored how reporters promoted the clash of minds while attempting to sway their audience to their side. A total of 20 news articles were selected randomly for the study.

8.4 Results

Collaboration Is the Solution

The journalists presented the news so that it was clear that collaboration among organisations was required to win the fight against doping. For example, Malidadi (2021) in an article titled "Mado, Government in Anti-Doping Project", published in *Times Group*, explains that the Malawi Anti-Doping Organisation (MADO) was set up to fight the malpractice by collaborating with the Malawi government. The article indicates a public function where the collaboration was publicly declared; the Malawi government was represented by the Minister of Sports, Ulemu Msungama.

Athletes and MADO have also shown signs of collaboration. In the article titled "Anti-Doping Body to Vet Athletes", Kambuwe (2020) posits that WADA has given MADO permission to begin conducting rigorous tests before athletes compete in any sports. The article illustrates high-level coordination not only among Malawi's top sporting organisations but also with WADA, a globally influential organisation.

Athletes and Their Officials Are Blank Slates

The papers also suggest that athletes and their authorities are unaware of anti-doping legislation and must be trained. For example, in the article "Lack of Knowledge Worries Anti-Doping Body", Sangala (2016) writes that the MADO board chairperson, James Mwenda, had indicated that most local athletes and officials lack doping knowledge. As a response, the organisation planned to launch a public awareness campaign to expose athletes and their officials to expertise so that they can be discouraged from using *"illegal performance-enhancing medicines."* Similarly, Mwenda contends that these stakeholders must understand that doping is a deadly *"enemy of sports"*. Chinoko (2016) argues that MADO had organised a major campaign that involved cycling, as well as radio, television, and newspaper commercials in both local languages and English.

Ironically, Sangala (2016) observes that most people do not know about anti-doping, and yet Kaoche et al. (2020, p. 7) argue that 77% of the athletes had a high level of anti-doping knowledge, and 22.1% had a medium level of awareness. Furthermore, these statements were made when Malawi seemed to be "clean" where all the 13 athletes drawn from football, netball, and boxing were tested for drugs and the results came out negative (Sangala, 2016).

This situation may make one wonder how the people who do not know about anti-doping were found to be "clean".

It can be argued that MADO targeted the 0.9% that did not have any knowledge of anti-doping and the 22.1% that had a medium level of knowledge. It can also be argued that MADO considered the knowledge levels low because it was only interested in Western doping methods and did not factor in indigenous doping methods rooted in *Juju*. Some individuals may not be aware of Western doping knowledge since Western doping is pricey and elite, yet doping is not a new concept in Malawi. In sports, there have always been examples of *Juju*, a form of doping.

The news reports and MADO leaned more towards a Western epistemic position that ignores and views African bodies as incapable of thinking. In these articles, MADO exhibited what Nyamnjoh (2017) refers to as African mimicry, in which African thinkers duplicate what the West claims and recreate as knowledge on African bodies to argue that Western epistemology is the only way of explaining African experiences.

Nyamnjoh (2017) believes that because Africans believe in the multiplicity of being, they reject these binary framings of African bodies. He uses Tutuola's argument that the human body is like a container that may exist in multiple ways. It can, for example, live in the human body, and when that person dies, the human soul can be inhibited by any other container, such as an animal or even a stone. Nyamnjoh (2017) adds that this kind of thinking shows that Africans are frontier thinkers who perceive reality from different angles, and they appreciate that people must be convivial thinkers who accommodate multiplicity of being. Conviviality can be extended to how the authors presented the articles, in that they could have considered the various ways in which doping is done. That is not to say that the Western conception of doping should be dismissed, but rather that it should be enriched by including different forms of doping that have been conceptualised in African knowledge systems.

Significantly, in this epistemic connection, Foucault (1995) also speaks on knowledge where he explains that many bodies have been incarcerated in that they are forced to embrace knowledge with which they are not even in agreement. The thinkers are trapped in a panoptic space where they believe that they are being monitored by the Western thinkers, resulting in governmentality and forcing them to accept the Western truth as the only truth. Thinkers must stand up and revolt against these normalised truths because they are a type of physical incarceration that is used to govern how people live their lives, reducing them to walking prisoners with chains around their brains (Foucault, 1995).

Athletes Are Childish

Athletes are also portrayed in Malawian sports media as young or childlike, needing sufficient guidance, caution, and discipline. For example, in the article titled "Anti-Doping Body Tips Flames Ahead of Afcon", Chirwa (2021) asserts that MADO had given advice to the Flames (Nickname for the Malawi National Men's Football Team) as they were approaching Africa Cup of Nations (Afcon) finals in Cameroon. The article shows that the advice given at an event was conducted by MADO Education Commission chairperson Oscar Kanjala and anti-doping education officer Yona Walesi. Flames team doctor Gift Ligomeka and Vice-captain John 'CJ' Banda expressed gratitude that the exercise was timely. Whether the counsel was helpful or not, it stands out that the athletes were viewed as children, in that they had to be warned against mischievous behaviour before allowing them to play. MADO authorities appear to have a patronising approach towards the athletes, similar to how a mother or father holds his or her child's hand and gives him or her advice before they go on vacation or to a new school. Just like a parent reprimanding a child, MADO is warning the child not to be mischievous, only that these athletes are not children and must be treated as adults who know what they want and can construct knowledge and rules of their being.

Athletes Are Crooks

Journalists sometimes portray athletes as crooks who can't be trusted. They are frequently suspected of doping, and that they normally get away with it because they are not tested at the local level. This framing, however, comes not only from the media but also from sports administrators who appear to have little faith in their own athletes. Manda (2014), in the article "FIFA Targets Tests on Chirambo, Kaipa", affirms that FIFA team arrived in Malawi without alerting the players that they would be tested for doping, thereby treating athletes like suspects or crooks who could not be trusted with the information that they would be examined. As a result, the players were antagonised and treated as lab specimens without a thinking brain, who were required to remain silent and wait for the results.

The athletes' previous behaviour of doping may have contributed to the suspicion. This situation raises the issue of profiling people, as athletes are no longer seen as individuals with unique perspectives on doping. They are all treated as suspects even if they haven't given the authorities any cause to distrust them. This means that the athletes have been reduced to sub-humans who are incapable of caring for their bodies and must thus be constantly scrutinised and subjected to conditions of war in which they are viewed as a potential enemy of sports, even though they have done nothing wrong previously (Chipeta, 2014).

One could claim that because the players consent to be tested at any moment by FIFA, they have no right to protest if tested unexpectedly. This reasoning may be correct; however, Owens (2011) cautions that determining whether consent was freely provided can be difficult. FIFA is a powerful organisation that oversees most of the world's major sporting events. If a player disagrees with them, they may be unable to compete in these key international events. Some sportsmen may grant their consent simply to be rid of FIFA, otherwise they would be suspected every day of their professional lives. On the other hand, FIFA is more than simply a body; it is a representative group of leaders from all around the world, including Africa, who make these decisions. As a result, the ideas may sometimes represent what the athlete's agents desire. This viewpoint may be correct, but these representatives are not athletes; instead, they are elites with elite experiences who have little understanding of what a day in the life of a runner in Malawi is like.

Similarly, *The Nation* (2012, April 16) in "Moyo awaits doping test results" shows that even though "Marathon king", Henry Moyohad won the 56 km 2012 Old Mutual Ultra Two Oceans Marathon, he could not receive his silver medal until the results of his anti-doping tests were received. One could argue that instead of waiting for the test before making the award, they should have made the award first and then retracted it if issues arose because the fact that they had to keep the prize from him rather shows how much they suspected his body of not being responsible. Although MADO places such a high value on anti-doping testing, Moyo claims that the tests are often difficult to interpret and that even athletes who do not dope aren't always sure if they took a banned substance before a race. For example, Moyo was stripped off his gold medal at the Kuala Lumpar Marathon in Malaysia in 2005 because the flu medicine he took prior to the race was confused for a banned substance. Apart from him, an anti-doping test failed a police officer from Zomba who was using flu medication, denying him the Kuala Lumpur Marathon gold and K1 million (*The Nation*, 2012, April 16). It is not surprising that Moyo passed the test, raising concerns on why he was considered guilty before being proven guilty (Manda, 2013). This unreliability of doping tests makes athletes fear FIFA, WADA, and MADO even when they have not done anything wrong, and in the process, they surrender their being to annihilation by these institutions that seem to own their bodies.

Malawi Doesn't Have Resources

In addition, the papers depict team doctors as unprofessional. In the article titled "FAM Challenges Team Doctors", Sangala (2017a) explains that Daud Suleman, a member of the Football Association of Malawi Executive Committee, voiced concern that team doctors were failing to supervise the health habits of their athletes, particularly those who were using performance-enhancing substances. Suleman argues that athletes' lives are becoming more complicated due to the foods and drinks they consume, which expose them to things on the banned list. As a result, the workshop produced specialised doping training for doctors. Twenty-five doctors attended the seminar, including several who work for Super League teams.

The reporters frequently highlight the absence of resources that can be used to determine whether or not the athletes are doping. In the article titled "No Lab Equipment to Check Athletes' Drug Use", Kaminjolo (2014) agrees that the lack of such a laboratory indicates that certain athletes in the country may cheat in games. From 2013 to 2016, MADO managed to test only 15 athletes from different sporting activities (Chinoko, 2016). The challenge can be observed across Southern Africa except South Africa; hence, athletes are only tested for anti-doping when participating in international games (Kaminjolo, 2014). As a result, MADO is appealing to funders to assist them in acquiring this costly but vital service locally. The author also explains why the founding of MADO is an important step forward in Malawi's anti-doping efforts. MADO is urging all sporting organisations to register with them, and MADO proposes that all athletes should be tested through the collection of samples that will be sent to South Africa for screening. However, the long-term solution is to persuade the government to come in and assist in the acquisition of the equipment (Kaminjolo, 2014).

The Law Is Prohibitive and Protective

The media also portrays anti-doping from a legal standpoint, implying that Malawian laws do not encourage clean sport. In the article titled "Anti-Doping Faces Legal Setback", Chinoko (2017) articulates that the refusal of Malawi's parliament to pass anti-doping legislation makes it harder to eradicate doping from the country. The reporter made these observations while covering an event hosted by MADO and attended by the Minister of Labour, Youth, Sports and Manpower Development Henry Mussa, representatives from the donor community, and athletes from various sporting disciplines and organisations. The event was intended to reveal Nyasa Big Bullets defender Yamikani Fodya and Blue Eagles Sisters centre Takondwa Lwazi as anti-doping ambassadors.

The other challenge is that some of the drugs that WADA bans do not fall under the Dangerous Drugs Act of Parliament. MADO is rendered powerless as a result of this circumstance, as it is unable to execute some WADA guidelines without breaching the constitution (Chinoko 2017). MADO can simply impose a ban, and no criminal proceedings can be carried out. This suggests that MADO didn't simply want to punish the athletes' sporting souls, which Foucault (1995) considered as the ultimate punishment, but they also wanted to punish the physical body. MADO would be perceived as advancing the oblivion of doping athletes' humanity.

MADO also wished that legislation could be enacted to provide it with parliamentary support and financing for its efforts. Chinoko (2017) points out that this was crucial because most of MADO's initiatives necessitate resources, and government assistance is desperately needed. MADO has made obligations such as building a laboratory to test the use of doping on players, but it cannot do so due to a lack of funding to obtain the costly technology.

However, one can argue that recognising MADO through the parliament does not guarantee that they will get sufficient government assistance. Many government institutions in Malawi, including the public hospital (Chipeta, 2014), are never adequately supported by the parliament in terms of money. Possibly it would just give MADO tools to annihilate athletes.

Oddly, MADO was lobbying for legislation that has already sparked controversy and been rejected by over 150,000 athletes across Europe. Why do they believe that the law will help Malawian athletes? It's hard to say why they think this contentious reform will work in Malawi, but one could surmise that MADO simply wants to maintain good relations with WADA and is dancing to every song that WADA is singing. WADA's proposed constitutional changes through MADO reveal that WADA doesn't just want to control MADO and athletes; it also wants to own the Malawi parliament when it comes to the Poisons Act.

Aside from that, the usage of the word "MALAWI" on the MADO acronym is unsupported by law. The Protected Flag, Emblems, and Names Act makes "Malawi" a protected name. The guilt of MADO also seems to be purged when the paper claims that MADO asked the Attorney General's Office for permission to use the protected name (Chinoko, 2017). The organisation is also enlisting the assistance of attorneys from the Attorney General's Office in drafting the legal framework. This raises the intriguing question of whether the application is only a formality or means anything at all, given that the same organisation they are applying to is also drafting the framework.

News organisations have also published on how journalists report on doping instances and how such reports must be carefully crafted. Kaminjolo (2016) in an article titled "MOC Tips Media on Anti-Doping Reporting" writes that the Malawi Olympic Committee (MOC) has cautioned journalists that inaccurate reporting on doping news could result in legal action. Because the matter is sensitive, MOC president Oscar Kanjala warned journalists that they have legal constraints on what they can and cannot write. As a result, they must obtain adequate training on how to expose doping. The instance of South African athlete Caster Semenya, who won enormous sums in legal battles due to poor reporting, is used by the MOC president to illustrate their position.

Bending the Will of Athletes

In the article "Anti-Doping Body to Vet Athletes", one can notice that Kambuwe (2020) attempts to persuade his or her audience that the vetting of athletes before their participation in the games is critical. He/she accomplishes this by subjecting the readers to dissonance where doping is perceived as drug abuse and thus not good for the body. The seriousness of substances in sports is also seen in the piece "FAM Challenges Team Doctors", where Sangala (2017a) explains that the use of performance-enhancing drugs is banned. This type of writing would impact players' behaviour since they would be afraid to consume it because if it were outlawed, any usage would result in significant consequences, such as being barred from participating in sports. Participating in sports is an enormous privilege, especially in a nation like Malawi, where sporting options are limited. As a result, there's a good chance that the threat may cause people to reconsider their decisions. Kalilombe (2019) shows how damaging the ban can be by relating the banning of Hellings Mwakasungula to anti-doping. As a result, MADO backed Mwakasungula's ban and exploited the situation to propagate anti-doping messages. MADO vice-general secretary Brutus Ndhlovu further explained that the banning should serve as a deterring event for other athletes who dope or are contemplating to start doping (Kalilombe, 2019). MADO justified its out-of-the-ordinary and *ultra-vias* behaviour by claiming that it promotes all forms of sportsmanship and opposes all forms of cheating, including betting and doping.

News reports also influence athletes' perceptions by making them believe that anti-doping is not being forced on them when it is. For example, Sangala (2016) argues that the athletes would be able to choose when they wish to engage in the anti-doping project by providing MADO with a calendar of activities. This involvement in the projects makes them feel like they are a part of the movement and gives them a sense of control over what happens. This allows individuals to easily accept the ideas thrust upon them and store them in their subconscious minds as well-thought-out, beneficial to them, and championed by themselves.

In the article, "No Lab Equipment to Check Athletes' Drug Use", Kaminjolo (2014) tries to influence change but not necessarily on the side of the athletes as it is always the case, but on the side of the government. He is urging the government to assist in acquiring much-needed testing facilities for the athletes. He accomplishes this by appealing to pity and demonstrating how the current status quo allows for cheating in local games. The article also shows that the only time athletes can be tested is when they attend international games, which means that the country has to seek help from South Africa, which might be costly and less efficient in the fight against doping.

MADO also provides anti-doping information to athletes as they prepare to leave for competitions. The athletes are usually ecstatic and eager to depart at this point. Taking advantage of this time to counsel the player is strategic in that they are already aware of the benefits of sports, particularly travel, and would not want to miss out on the opportunity, necessitating the need to listen carefully and attentively. For example, in the article "Anti-Doping Body Tips Flames Ahead of Afcon", Chirwa (2021) explains that MADO gave a health talk to the Flames when they were ready for the Afcon. This indicated that the MADO message had been accompanied by some form of positive reinforcement, creating an ideal setting in which the participants may be persuaded. Reminding them before the games would also provide them with new information as they prepare for big tournaments (Chirwa, 2021).

Furthermore, athletes should not believe that they would be able to quit doping when the games are close, as FIFA will catch them off guard. Manda (2014), in the article "FIFA Targets Tests on Chirambo, Kaipa", writes that FIFA had tested Douglas Chirambo and Bongani Kaipa to ensure they were not doping. The coverage of this story emphasised the importance of athletes remaining drug-free in their sport because if they use drugs in local games and then clean up when international competitions approach, they may be caught by surprise. Football Association of Malawi (FAM) Chief Executive Officer Suzgo Nyirenda also indicated that they were not informed of the coming of FIFA officials who were accompanied by Dr Mathews Mangondo (Manda, 2014). The players were on their own in this scenario, and the only thing that could save them was being clean.

Kambuwe (2020) further explains that WADA, which is an international organisation, is also worried about the state of affairs. The use of an international organisation is an emotional trigger in most Malawians who experienced colonial domination, as this might be seen to undermine the ability of the local people to solve their problems. The use of colonial tendencies to influence perception may also be seen in an interview with the president of Malawi's boxing association. The writer also attempts to sway perceptions by assigning human beings to ranks, with those who appear to be more human beings being heard and treated seriously. The writer uses this narrative to introduce authority in his report, placing humans on some hierarchy, much as white people did during colonial times when those in power were more human than the subjects.

The continued hierarchy of being demonstrates the extent to which whiteness persists in Malawi. Whiteness, a privilege, is rooted in the desire to rank human bodies. Being white or black is not determined by skin colour; race has no bearing on skin colour. It has to do with privilege. This is why the black consciousness thinkers claimed that a black person is any person who has experienced suffering because of their skin colour. All black people who have collaborated with white people automatically lose their blackness (Biko, 1971). Nyamnjoh (2012) observes that in most countries whiteness does not seem to be obvious because most people do not have light skin that is associated with privilege and whiteness. Just like in the times of Steve Biko, there are still other Malawians who have collaborated with whiteness, and their whiteness can be seen in their everyday life. This is why people sometimes describe their friends as white because they enjoy privileges. Black people, collaborating with coloniality to accumulate privileges for themselves, forfeit their blackness.

Challenging whiteness in Malawi would not mean "whiteness" for everyone because, in the end, it is unrealistic that everyone would enjoy white privilege. But it is possible to unsettle whiteness and create an equitable country. Whiteness can be unsettled using conviviality where people from all walks of life can meet and share ideas (Nyamnjoh, 2017). In this way, the news reporters would become convivial centres, and they will not always be interviewing people of influence. They would also interview the athletes and the general Malawian populace. The interviews would not just be symbolic to window dress multiplicity of voices, but the ordinary people would also be viewed as authorities on issues that affect their lives and would not be objectified by elite and Western thinkers or their African mimics.

A Crush of Mind and Souls

The use of dissonance can also be noticed through the crush of minds that the journalists employ. In the article "Anti-Doping Body to Vet Athletes", the crush of mind can be noticed when Kambuwe (2020) writes that the president of the Malawi Boxing Association has already approved the request that the athletes be vetted. Using such an influential leader was intended to persuade other leaders to accept the concept because their minds had been crushed into believing that they should not be left behind because other powerful Malawian leaders might have already received the progress.

At the same time, the athletes are being mentally primed to embrace the proposition because the writer has shown that their leaders have already agreed. Athletes frequently battle to be included in national events, and such initiatives are driven to a greater extent by sports management, who have a greater say in who gets to play. Players must accept this endorsed effort to participate. It's worth noting that there was no appeal to logic in this mental crush. No attempt was made to explain to the audience why the project is beneficial to game fairness or human bodies. They state that using drugs is abuse at one point, but they do not detail why this is so. The writer was more concerned with shattering the audience's emotions to sway them to their viewpoint.

MADO has also been known to use athletes to promote their anti-doping messages. For example, in the article "Yamikani Fodya, Takondwa Lwazi Unveiled as Clean-Sports Ambassadors", Sangala (2017b) writes that Nyasa Big Bullets defender Yamikani Fodya and Blue Eagles Sisters player Takondwa Lwazi are clean players. This knowledge was significant because it demonstrated that if these talented athletes did not utilise drugs to enhance their abilities, other athletes could remain clean and thriving. MADO even invited politicians like Henry Mussa, the Minister of Labour, Youth, Sports and Manpower Development, to the opening event at Bingu International Stadium to get more people to watch the promotion.

In the article "FAM Challenges Team Doctors", Sangala (2017a) also uses an influential figure to crush the minds of his audience. He mentions Daud Suleman, a member of the FAM Executive Committee, as saying that doping was condemned. Because influential people are engaged in the issue, this strategy will cause participants to take the issue seriously. Because influential people can use their authority to punish and reprimand individuals who do not do what they want, athletes may be convinced to change their behaviour, especially when sporting opportunities are few in Malawi. The use of influential names is also seen where he mentions that the doctors would be trained by former Flames doctor Mangondo who was trained by FIFA and current Flames doctor Levison Mwale. FIFA is an international organisation and governs football across the globe. The fact that such an organisation taught Mangondo may convey that he is well versed in the subject and should be treated seriously in his appeals to authorities. By including contemporary frames, the journalists create a professional undertone that encourages participants to listen and take the conversations seriously.

In places where athletes and sports officials are made to regard themselves as less informed, the article's crush of mind can be felt. This claim causes dissonance in the athletes and officials, who wonder what they don't know, and this dissonance promotes a desire to learn – thus, they are willing to participate in the activities.

The fact that FIFA can just fly into the nation creates a state of mind in which the players are constantly concerned about being detected if they use drugs. Manda (2014), in the article "FIFA Targets Tests on Chirambo, Kaipa", argues that unexpected visits are a common tendency, as Chirambo says he was not startled when FIFA came with their surprise visit because he recalls a similar visit while he was playing for the Under-17 and Under-20 national teams. FIFA gives the athletes the impression that they are in a panoptic realm where their entire professional life is being monitored. This is a form of Foucauldian punishment and discipline where players are controlled and punished when they disobey.

Another mind-numbing approach employed by media is to refer to anti-doping sport as "clean sport". The phrase is used to describe a situation where one does not use performance-enhancing substance. However, elites and people of influence have other ways of enhancing their performance, which is out of reach for most poor athletes. The phrase "clean sport" therefore controls the poor athletes from enhancing their bodies as their rich counterparts explore options that do not involve substances but do work. For example, people from privileged countries are psychologically prepared to look at themselves as superior over those from developing countries because they have the best sporting equipment and counselling services. As such, each time athletes from developing countries play against athletes from rich countries, they are already psychologically defeated, while those that come from rich countries are already psychologically enhanced. The psychological enhancement produces chemicals/hormones that demonstrate how inequality can be so dirty and can push the Othered bodies into continued failure in international sport.

8.5 Conclusion

According to the findings of this study, anti-doping news coverage in Malawi portrays the anti-doping effort as a complex battle that can only be won through collaboration. This gives the readers a positive impression of anti-doping. However, the anti-doping news frequently depicts athletes as immature, criminals, and illiterate. This is problematic because it projects athletes in a negative light, even though these pictures are based on profiling and whiteness. Whiteness and profiling must be addressed because they create a hierarchy of being in which athletes appear to be second-class citizens, with MADO and WADA claiming ownership of their bodies. These depictions evoke unpleasant emotional reactions in a country like Malawi, which has a tragic history. The reports also appear to support the West's understanding of doping. Traditional methods, including *Juju*, are frequently ignored. This could be because Western epistemology regards *Juju* as a superstition, something that is only imagined and that its actuality must be challenged.

The study also revealed that media try to sway players by urging them not to take drugs when the game is near, frightening them with an unannounced FIFA visit, and giving them the impression that anti-doping is their idea. Anti-doping is also associated with powerful people, making it difficult for people to reject the information. Successful athletes are often used to deceive unsuccessful athletes and their managers into believing that they don't know enough about the subject to pursue it. Finally, although it is related to disparities, anti-doping is portrayed as a clean sport. These techniques of influencing the audience seem to downplay reasoning so that the audience can accept anti-doping without adequately understanding what anti-doping is and why they must refrain from it.

References

Banfi, G., Lombardi, G., Colombini, A., & Lippi, G. (2010). A world apart: inaccuracies of laboratory methodologies in anti-doping testing. *Clinica Chimica Acta, 411*(15), 1003–1008. https://doi.org/10.1016/j.cca.2010.03.039

Biko, S. (1971). The definition of black consciousness. Deep Green Resistance News Service. https://dgrnewsservice.org/resistance-culture/anti-racism/the-definition-of-black-consciousness-december-1971-south-africa/

Bryman, A. (1988). *Quantity and Quality in Social Research*. London: Unwin Hayman.

Chinoko, C. (2016, February 7). Anti-doping body to intensify awareness. *The Nation Online*. www.mwnation.com/anti-doping-body-to-intensify-awareness/

Chinoko, C. (2017, March 2). Anti-doping faces legal setback. *The Nation Online*. www.mwnation.com/anti-doping-faces-legal-setback/

Chipeta, J. B. (2014). Factors that affect staff morale in tertiary hospitals in Malawi: a case study of Kamuzu Central Hospital. *Journal of Human Resource and Sustainability Studies, 2*(04), Article 04. https://doi.org/10.4236/jhrss.2014.24024

Chirwa, G. (2021, December 24). Anti-doping body tips Flames ahead of Afcon. *The Nation Online*. www.mwnation.com/?p=325003

Communication, I., & Social. (2012, November 26). Cognitive Dissonance Theory – Real Life Examples. *Communication Theory*. Accessed 18th of April 2023 www.communicationtheory.org/cognitive-dissonance-theory/

Creswell, J. W., Hanson, W. E., & Plano, C. (2007). Qualitative research designs; selection and implementation. *The Counseling Psychologist*, 35(2), 236–264.

Fairhurst, G. T., & Sarr, R. A. (1996). The art of framing: managing the language of leadership. https://3lib.net/book/18022602/397c42

Foucault, M. (1995). *Discipline and Punish: The Birth of Prison*. Toronto: Random House.

Framing Theory. (2011, March 17). Mass communication theory. Accessed 18th of April 2023. https://masscommtheory.com/theory-overviews/framing-theory/

Framing Theory. (2012, November 1). Communication Studies. www.communicationstudies.com/communication-theories/framing-theory

Kalilombe, F. (2019, May 17). Body applauds FIFA on Mwakasungula ban. *The Nation Online*. www.mwnation.com/body-applauds-fifa-on-mwakasungula-ban/

Kambuwe, M. (2020, October 27). Anti-doping body to Vet athletes—*The Times Group Malawi*. https://times.mw/anti-doping-body-to-vet-athletes/

Kaminjolo, S. (2014, December 20). No lab equipment to check athletes drug use. *The Nation Online*. www.mwnation.com/no-lab-equipment-check-athletes-drug-use/

Kaminjolo, S. (2016, February 14). MOC tips media on anti-doping reporting. *The Nation Online*. www.mwnation.com/moc-tips-media-on-anti-doping-reporting/

Kaoche, J. M. C. (2019). *Evaluation of Knowledge and Attitudes on Doping by Football Athletes, Coaches and Sponsors in Malawi*. Kenyatta University.

Kaoche, J. M. C., Rintaugu, E. G., Kamenju, J., & Mwangi, F. M. (2020). Knowledge on doping among football athletes, coaches and sponsors in Malawi. *Journal of Physical Education and Sport Management, 11*(2), 5–13. https://doi.org/10.5897/JPESM2020.0346

Kovač, U. (2016, October 28). "Juju" and "Jars": how African athletes challenge western notions of doping. *The Conversation*. http://theconversation.com/juju-and-jars-how-african-athletes-challenge-western-notions-of-doping-67567

Malidadi, M. (2021, October 5). Mado, government in anti-doping project. *The Times Group Malawi*.times.mw/mado-government-in-anti-doping-project/

Manda, S. (2013, July 5). Moyo passes doping test. *The Nation Online*. www.mwnation.com/moyo-passes-doping-test/

Manda, S. (2014, January 30). FIFA targets tests on Chirambo, Kaipa. *The Nation Online*. www.mwnation.com/fifa-targets-tests-on-chirambo-kaipa/

McCombs, M. E., Shaw, D. L., & Weaver, D. H. (2014). New directions in agenda-setting theory and research. *Mass Communication and Society, 17*, 781–802.

Møller, V. (2014). Who guards the guardians? *The International Journal of the History of Sport, 31*(8), 934–950. https://doi.org/10.1080/09523367.2013.826652

Mwangi, S. (2018). *Role of the Media in Curbing Doping among Middle and Long-Distance Runners in Kenya* (Master's Thesis). University of Nairobi, Kenya

Njororai, W. W. S. (2019). *Culture of Magic and Sorcery in African Football in Africa's Elite Football*. London: Routledge.

Ntaba, J. M. (2012). Negotiating family planning radio messages among Malawian rural men of traditional authority Kadewere, Chiradzulo district. https://commons.ru.ac.za/vital/access/manager/Repository/vital:3548?site_name=Rhodes%20University&view=null&f0=sm_type%253A%2522text%2522&f1=sm_type%253A%2522Thesis%2522&sort=null&f2=sm_creator%253A%2522Ntaba%252C+Jolly+Maxwell%2522&f3=sm_type%253A%2522Masters%2522

Nyamnjoh, F. B. (2012). Blinded by sight: divining the future of anthropology in Africa. *Africa Spectrum, 3*(2/3), 63–92.

Nyamnjoh, F. B. (2019, July 9). ICTs as Juju: African inspiration for understanding the compositeness of being human through digital technologies. *Journal of African Media Studies, 11*(3), 27–291.

Nyamnjoh, F. B. N. (2017). Incompleteness: Frontier Africa and the currency of conviviality. *Journal of Asian and African Studies, 52*(3), 253–270.

Owens, D. (2011). The possibility of consent. *Ratio: An International Journal of Analytical Philosophy, 24*(4), 402–421. https://doi.org/10.1111/j.1467-9329.2011.00509.x

Sangala, T. (2016, February 8). Lack of knowledge worries anti-doping body. *The Times Group Malawi*. https://times.mw/lack-of-knowledge-worries-anti-doping-body/

Sangala, T. (2017a). FAM challenges team doctors. https://times.mw/fam-challenges-team-doctors/

Sangala, T. (2017b, March 2). Yamikani Fodya, Takondwa Lwazi unveiled as clean-sport ambassadors. https://times.mw/yamikani-fodya-takondwa-lwazi-unveiled-as-clean-sport-ambassadors/

The Nation. (2012, April 16). Moyo awaits doping test results. *The Nation Online*. Available at www.mwnation.com/moyo-awaits-doping-test-results/

Uroš, K. (2016). *Football dreams, Pentecostalism and migration in Southwest Cameroon*. Amsterdam: Global Sport Blog. https://global-sport.eu

Vipene, J. B. (2003). Vipene J.B. and Amasiatu, N. (2003). drug abuse in sports and its psychological effects on athletes: sports biomechanics. *Journal of Vocational, Science and Educational Development (JOVSED), 4*, 66–71.

World Anti-Doping Agency. (2022). Media. World Anti-Doping Agency. /www.wada-ama.org/en/media

Chapter 9

Research-Based Educational Approach and Doping Management

Charles Nyasa, Blessings Kaunda-Khangamwa, and Enock Chisati

9.1 Introduction

Doping in sports refers to athletes' use or attempted use of illicit substances to enhance athletic performance (Bird et al., 2016; Kaoche, 2019). It is a global problem rooted in ancient history (Bahrke and Yasalis, 2002; Dorota and Derman, 2016). The use of doping agents in sports is prohibited worldwide. This is due to the detrimental effects that performance-enhancing substances (PES) pose on athletes' health, equality in sport (fair play), and the spirit of Olympism, which entails the ethical pursuit of human excellence through true perfection of natural talents (Kaoche, 2019; World Anti-Doping Agency [WADA], 2021). For this reason, WADA was established in 1999 to coordinate the fight against doping worldwide through the World Anti-Doping Programme [WADP] (Bird et al., 2016; Kaoche et al., 2020; WADA, 2021). At the national level, the WADP is administered by national anti-doping organisations.

WADA operations and the WADP administration may be understood as encompassing three primary functions: doping prevention, anti-doping rule enforcement, and quality assurance. The anti-doping Code, international standards, and best-practice models serve to ensure global harmonisation of anti-doping efforts by supplying consistent regulations across all sports organisations and national authorities (Canadian Centre for Ethics in Sports, 2022) and set the basis for doping control and enforcement activities to facilitate detection and deterrence (European Commission, 2014). On the other hand, the programme's prevention strategies are designed to inform athletes about the biological and disciplinary repercussions of doping, extol the virtue of playing true, and enhance frontline familiarisation with up-to-date prohibited lists (European Commission, 2014; Gatterer et al., 2020). According to Article 2 of the Code, responsibility rests upon the athlete to know what constitutes a rule violation and substances or methods that are listed as prohibited. Ignorance of these substances or methods is not an excuse (WADA, 2021).Education is one of the prevention strategies that not only serves to raise awareness of elements of the Code but also helps instil values and

DOI: 10.4324/9781003370796-11

develop behaviours that foster and protect the spirit of sport (WADA, 2021). With intentional and unintentional doping on the rise (Shibata et al., 2017), it is considered a fundamental principle that an athlete's first experience with anti-doping is through education rather than through doping control (WADA, 2021). Quality control, a third function of the programme, involves using science and research to improve detection methods' understanding, accuracy, and feasibility. Recently, WADA has been interested in social science research to understand the human factor and sociocultural elements that influence doping behaviour.

In terms of extent, reports show that doping instances are rising globally, and this is despite all earlier efforts (Johnson, 2011). Currently, the global prevalence of doping is pegged at 1–2% based on doping control testing data and 1–70% based on questionnaire-based surveys, with significant inter-discipline and inter-nation variations in both cases (de Hon et al., 2014; Kaoche et al., 2020). For instance, estimates as high as 6.6% and 16% have been reported among football players in Italy and Cameroon, respectively (Kaoche, 2019). Faiss et al. (2020) found an overall blood doping prevalence of 18% in a 2011 cohort of track and field athletes at the World Athletics Championship and 15% in a 2013 cohort of a similar event. In 2015, Al Ghobain et al. (2016) reported a 4.3% survey-based doping prevalence among Saudi athletes from various disciplines. Meanwhile, a more extensive 2020 study of the same population group reported a 2.24% prevalence using doping control testing (Aljaloud et al., 2020), thus reflecting an obvious under-detection problem among studies based on laboratory testing data. Therefore, it can be implied that the actual global prevalence of doping may be higher than what is often reported in the literature. A 2014 review of numbers and methods reported a 14–39% global prevalence of intentional doping among elite athletes using a more plausible randomised responses technique involving questionnaires and models of biological parameters (de Hon et al., 2014).

This chapter proposes developing evidence-based research to generate baseline data to inform the design and implementation of a culturally responsive anti-doping educational programme for athletes and athlete support personnel in Malawi and allow its evaluation. Malawi is chosen as a point of reference because of its underdeveloped sport systems, scanty literature on the topic, and a culturally pinned drug use context which closely characterise most non-Western resource-limited nations. Because of this, a review of literature and programmes in geographically underfunded southern African countries and the global north was conducted to understand ways of promoting clean sport and developing effective programmes for all. From the outset, the chapter highlights the need for anti-doping education and research in Malawi. Then it illuminates the systemic model of doping behaviour as a guiding theoretical framework of choice, considering its contextual fit over contemporary frameworks. In the end, a discussion on the operationalisation of the model to guide the design and implementation of anti-doping research and education in Malawi is presented with a rigorously crafted example.

9.2 Malawi's Doping Landscape

Malawi signed the Copenhagen Declaration on Anti-Doping in Sport in 2003 and later ratified the United Nations Educational, Scientific and Cultural Organization (UNESCO) International Convention against Doping in Sport. In 2013 the Malawi Anti-Doping Organisation (MADO) was formed as a national level anti-doping body (Kaoche et al., 2020). As of 2020, WADA had approved MADO's proposal to adopt local regulations which showed commitment to intensify anti-doping efforts beginning the year 2021 (Chinoko, 2016). This was followed by appeals for stakeholder support to augment MADO's efforts through facilitation of infrastructural development to ease domestic testing, and surveys to establish baseline data for use when framing social science research and awareness projects.

It is no secret that Malawi still faces challenges implementing the preventative and doping control aspects of the anti-doping Code. There is also a general paucity of information on how the WADP is and ought to be administered locally. Similarly, data on the extent at which doping is practised, the forms that it takes, and the role of frontline personnel in both amateur and elite sport is scarce, making evaluation of past and present anti-doping efforts hardly possible. A critical analysis of Malawi's anti-doping efforts reveals challenges related to local prevalence data, social science research, and enforcement of rules.

Shortage of Prevalence Data

Doping prevalence is one of the reliable parameters for determining the extent of doping and gauging the success of anti-doping efforts in any locality. However, it is a difficult parameter to measure systematically (de Hon et al., 2014). This is because the practice itself is contextual and occurs varyingly across settings. In addition to that, the lack of uniformity in data collection methodologies across settings, challenges at testing every athlete, and preference for self-reported surveys lead to underestimation of pooled figures for establishing the overall prevalence of such a prohibited and often undisclosed practice.

There is evidence that the southern African region suffers a shortage of data on the prevalence of doping, with available sources originating from self-reported questionnaire surveys and very few actual testing exercises (Sagoe et al., 2014). This presents a technical problem as these studies cannot talk to each other and their results can hardly be infused to give a unified conclusion. A meta-analysis of studies published from 1970 to 2013, for instance, reported a 2.4% lifetime prevalence of anabolic androgen steroid use in

African sports (Sagoe et al., 2014). Meanwhile, similar country-specific studies have reported such higher prevalence as 3.8% in Ghana (Sagoe et al., 2015); 3.9% in South Africa (Gradidge et al., 2011); and 5.5% in Nigeria (Sagoe et al., 2014). There is limited data for Malawi.

The relative scarcity of data in Malawi is due to limitations in testing coupled with the rarity of high-quality research studies on the subject, and not due to the absence of doping cases. There is plenty of anecdotal evidence of doping practices among elite and amateur Malawian athletes. A recent pilot study of elite football players from Malawi's top league found a PES use prevalence of 91% (Chisati et al., 2022). Moreover, the recent upward trend in attention accorded local anti-doping efforts shows that doping is a growing reality and a worrisome issue even to the country's sport authorities (Chinoko, 2016). A cross-sectional study by Kaoche (2019) found that of the 235 Malawian athletes who did not use PES, 1.7% were aware of those teammates who did. A further 4.2% of athlete support personnel were aware of doping instances that took place in their teams, while 46.7% of football sponsors knew some athletes who doped (Kaoche, 2019). Overall, the scarcity of doping prevalence data in Malawi has obscured the extent of the doping problem, limited adaptability of international standards and best-practice models, and continues to frustrate development of new programmes from scratch.

Scarcity of Social Science Research

Knowledge may shape one's attitude towards a conduct. Attitudes in turn build onto perceptions which, together with a person's behavioural, normative, as well as control beliefs, pose a direct effect on doping behaviour (or doping intention) (Dorota and Derman, 2016; WADA, 2021). According to Ajzen's theory of planned behaviour (TBC), volitional human behaviour is a function of the intention to perform the behaviour, and intention is hypothesised to be a function of attitudes, subjective norms, and perceived behavioural control (Sniehotta et al., 2014). Meanwhile, Whitaker and colleagues (2014) admit that research employing TBC has largely and successfully proven that attitudes and social norms emerge as predictors of doping behaviour through mediator intentions.

So far, the few studies on the roles of various personnel in the fight against doping in Malawi have produced mixed results and little is known on what aspects of the Code athletes and significant others really know (Kaoche, 2019; Kaoche et al., 2020). As a result, not much can be said on prevailing attitudes towards anti-doping in Malawi let alone the factors that may have driven adoption of those attitudes. A cross-sectional study on evaluation of doping knowledge and attitudes in Malawi found that over 23%, 54%, and 40% of athletes, coaches, and sponsors, respectively, had medium to low levels of knowledge regarding doping elements, and fellow players were an important source of anti-doping information of all significant others within an athlete's circle (Kaoche, 2019). Attitude towards anti-doping was also scored poorly with 25% of athletes and 40% of sponsors registering medium to low levels of the attribute (Kaoche, 2019). Further analysis of the study showed a few ambiguities in participants' reporting, particularly where only 100 athletes reported to have ever been tested for doping yet 214 indicated to have been tested once. This is confusing but not surprising in self-reported baseline surveys and stresses the need to frame survey questions carefully. Additionally, knowledge of doping needs to be considered in its broad terminological sense as comprising awareness of both the prohibited list and processes of the WADP. Chebet (2014) employed the term more broadly in a study of elite Kenyan athletes.

Enforcement Challenges

Anti-doping is as much an institutional mandate as it is a personal one. Institutions (organisations or bodies) are vital in enforcing elements of the Code by delivering doping control and quality assurance functions of the WADP. For this reason, Article 12 of the Code empowers signatories to sanction any organisation under their authority that does not follow, uphold, implement, and enforce the Code within their area of competence (WADA, 2021). Although noticeable steps have been taken by Malawi towards honouring its commitment to the Code (mostly through stakeholder sensitisation and sample submission for testing), little has been done to create or empower institutions to administer elements of the Code locally and most efficiently. Apart from instituting MADO as a national anti-doping entity, there has been little effort to accredit laboratories and ease local testing of athletes. Similarly, Malawian media houses have been silent on anti-doping issues as there are no long-term nationally institutionalised anti-doping awareness programmes, and the potential of existing academic institutions to support testing, research, and educational abilities still is untapped. In 2013, with support from UNESCO, MADO held a sensitisation training session that was attended by 30 sport administrators and health experts (Nyasa Times, 2013). However, this number was too small to quench the educational and awareness needs of the nation's entire sport fraternity.

Overall, the scarcity of reliable evidence and data on doping prevalence, practices, and associated attitudes among athletes and supporting personnel in Malawi threatens compliance to the Code, mocks existing efforts, and slows promotion of clean-sport behaviours. Although researchers have tried to evaluate doping prevalence before, the lack of comprehensive and sustainable national testing programmes (and therefore the lack of dependable data) has made arrival at exact figures a challenge. This has led some into estimating prevalence through self-reports (Kaoche, 2019). However, such studies have depended on the assumption that people were aware of basic elements of the Code, prohibited lists, and the anti-doping programme itself, which was not the case. It has already been said that the educational programmes so far delivered by MADO since 2013 are too few to cater for the growing local sport fraternity. Therefore, there is a definite need for mass educational programmes to raise awareness on elements of the WADP and to provoke values that people may have on the furtherance of clean sport. To succeed, such programmes need to be built upon existing knowledge, and account for the forms, attitudes, and contextual factors that surround doping and anti-doping in Malawian communities, which are also not well known. Luckily, there is a way to address these two deficits concurrently and action research that adopts a bottom-up approach is the answer.

9.3 Theoretical and Conceptual Frameworks

The use of drugs in sport has been subjected to increased theoretical critique over the years. Sociologists, psychologists, and other academics often frame research on biomedical and psychosocial aspects of doping basing upon various theoretical constructs (Morente-Sánchez and Zabala, 2013). For instance, earlier sociological studies often used a single theory to understand or explain complex doping behaviours at the level of the athlete. These included the theories of planned behaviour, reasoned action, social cognitive, self-determination, as well as triadic influence (Backhouse et al., 2015; Sniehotta et al., 2014). These theories have thus been the basis for earlier anti-doping programmes. However, Woolway et al. (2020) advised that since anti-doping programmes tend to target diverse cultures, their design must consider not only individuals but also methodical, logistical, and theoretical issues often at play. Moreover, the problem of drug abuse occurs both within and outside the settings of sport. As such, Connor and Mazanov (2009) advocate looking at personal, social, and historical issues when applying sociological theories to illuminate forces that drive doping in sport.

Recent developments in sport psychology have shown that doping behaviour results from both rational and irrational forces (Backhouse et al., 2015; Gibbons et al., 1998; Johnson, 2011). Rational forces are those goal-oriented processes that follow a logical sequence leading to decision-making (behavioural intention), while irrational forces refer to reactive deliberate processes that modulate decisions to engage in a particular behaviour (behavioural willingness), in this case doping (Gibbons et al., 1998; Whitaker et al., 2014). However, an individual's perceived likelihood to perform the behaviour (behavioural expectation) is said to rely on opportunity, previous behaviour or habits, and alternative behaviours available, among other factors (Gibbons et al., 1998), which often bring discussion on the role of sociopolitical factors in PES use among athletes. Thus, several factors influence doping in sport (Kaoche, 2019).

It may be argued that most studies on PES use in Africa have often looked at the doping problem through the lenses of Western culture. This is unsurprising considering that most foundational theories originated from the west and have been appraised within Western sociopolitical contexts. As a result, African research investigating the link between knowledge, attitudes, and behaviours in relation to doping quickly subscribed to the behaviourist model (Chebet, 2014; Muwonge et al., 2015; Shibata et al., 2017). Without referring to flaws associated with this link (Gibbons et al., 1998; Ogden, 2015; Sniehotta et al., 2014), the obvious sociocultural differences across settings entail that doping in southern Africa at least may possess a different trajectory that is rooted in beliefs, culture, and context-specific constructs which may best be represented by wider-spanning contemporary models (Kabiri et al., 2019; Woolway et al., 2020). As such, a top-down research approach in these settings may be detrimental to comprehensive exploration of the problem and long-term carryover. To date, studies employing multi-theoretical or multi-level frameworks in southern Africa remain scarce. It is highly probable, therefore, that anti-doping educational programmes so far delivered in Malawi lacked sound adaptation to the local context.

9.4 The Need for Research-Based Anti-Doping Education

The evolving nature of anti-doping rules, international guidelines, and best-practice models, coupled with the evolution of our understanding of theoretical bases of learning, prevention, as well as behaviour change require adoption of admirably adapted and evidence-based anti-doping strategies. These strategies must be tested and proven to work in local environments within affordable cost limits. This chapter acknowledges the need for anti-doping awareness and education in Malawi and proposes development of evidence-based research to generate baseline data leading to the design of a culturally responsive anti-doping educational programme for Malawian athletes and athlete support personnel. Evidence generated through such research will also aid development of adapted detection programmes and strengthen enforcement institutions.

While acknowledging the many theories that explain knowledge-attitude-perception-beliefs as well as PES use experiences among athletes and supporting personnel (Backhouse et al., 2015), this chapter moves to recommend application of the systemic model of doping behaviour (updated as systemic socio-cognitive perspective) by Johnson (2011, 2012) to guide development of culturally responsive anti-doping projects. The systemic model is based on Bronfenbrenner's (1977, 1979, 2001) bio-ecological theory of human development and Bandura's (1986) social learning theory and posits that doping behaviour is influenced by one's environment (i.e. social causation), his or her genetic makeup (i.e. social selection), and a complex interaction between these and the social context (Gibbons et al., 1998; Johnson, 2011). This model's unique position on the interaction between an individual's subjectively perceived experiences, his or her environment, and the prevalent social context has potential to afford such a grassroots research project, as this is a more exploratory space to successfully inform development of new anti-doping programmes. Moreover, the scarcity of baseline data on doping in Malawi necessitates the use of research frameworks that are wide spanning.

The systemic model of doping behaviour by Johnson (2011) illustrates an interaction between a person's subjectively perceived experiences and his environment. These experiences include thoughts, feelings, and behaviours which depend on the person's genotype that is acquired from his or her biological parents at conception (i.e. social selection). In the model, the person and his or her parents are defined with dashed lines to emphasise that the person–environment barrier is permeable. Meanwhile, environmental factors are seen to continually influence one's behaviours (i.e. social causation). In addition, a person's doping behaviour (i.e. either doping or not doping) is said to affect the person and the environment directly in a reciprocal fashion. Changes over time (e.g. epigenesis and development) also play a role.

In the application of the systemic model, the proposed research projects will need to consider variations in individuals' social selection (feelings, perceptions, beliefs, age, and attitudes), their environment (culture, history, socio-economic status, peers, and governing bodies), and related social factors (expectations, acceptance, reinforcers, and rewards) as bases for explaining doping attitudes, beliefs, and behaviours among athletes and athlete support personnel. One of the primary goals of such projects would therefore be to consider how these constructs of the systemic model, subjected to investigation, are useful in informing development of a culturally responsive national anti-doping awareness programme aimed at imparting knowledge, enriching attitudes, and shaping social skills.

The second and more direct objective of the proposed research would be to understand the precise factors that drive doping among Malawian athletes, as guided by the model. This can be carried out in three steps, starting with a baseline study to illuminate the context and provoke existing values and perceptions. After this, an implementation exercise to develop awareness packages and a pilot educational programme can follow. The last step would involve evaluating the impact of the pilot programme leading to validation, upgrading, and retesting. Table 9.1 illustrates how various constructs of the systemic model can be applied in practice to inform design of baseline research leading to development of a culturally responsive anti-doping educational programme for Malawi.

Table 9.1 Illustration of application of the systemic model and socio-cognitive theory to the design of baseline research and educational programmes

Components and constructs of the model	*Elements of the constructs*	*Considerations during baseline research*	*Considerations during educational package development and piloting*
Components of schema that shape athletes' doping decisions and behaviour	Relevance to own goals Personal meaningfulness Ability to dope (i.e. access or opportunity) Ability to self-regulate (i.e. evade detection systems)	Include assessment of knowledge of performance enhancement (its history in local context), PES use, role of MADO, and healthier alternatives Assess attitudes, perception, exposure or affordability of PES, and strength of institutions	Include materials addressing healthier alternatives and their enablers Focus on harmful effects of doping Involve athletes in long-term community drug avoidance programmes Highlight consequences of a positive result
Important environmental factors that affect doping behaviour	Motivational climate (social expectation) Peer and cultural norms Environmental (social) influencers Reinforcers	Obtain an overview of communities' perceptions on sport, athletes, winning, doping, and drug abuse Assess local historical and cultural landscape in relation to doping Assess understanding of roles of supporting personnel in anti-doping	Include a public statement of every participant's commitment to clean sport Train athlete support personnel separately and comprehensively Attach some reward (e.g. certificate)
Important individual (personal) factors that shape doping behaviour	Developmental stage (cognitive, psychosocial, as well as socio-emotional) Personality factors Perceptions and beliefs Ego and process orientation	Stratify participants with respect to age range and sporting level Use hypothetical situations to gain insights on personality and other intrinsic factors Tailor research questions to historical contexts Employ proper research designs	Stratify participants with respect to age range and sporting level Include socials skills development components (e.g. mentorship, parental guidance, peer, and expert support) Instil facts and debunk contextual myths

The Role of Schemas in Doping Decisions

In psychology, schemas are higher-order cognitive functions that underlie many aspects of human knowledge and skills (Brewer and Nakamura, 1984). Bartlett (1932) defined a schema as an active organisation of past reactions or past experiences, which must always be supposed to be operating in any well-adapted organic response. They serve as frameworks that help one understand and interpret information, thereby forming the basis of how one relates with the world. Applying the concept to doping behaviour, Johnson posits that schemas involving decisions and behaviours consist of an individual's subjective perceptions of consequences of doping (regardless of whether desirable or not), likelihood of the consequences occurring, and the role of pertinent environmental factors (Johnson, 2012). Table 9.1 shows elements of schemas that may shape an athlete's perception towards doping and whether they may end up doping. For instance, a person must first be able to attach meaningfulness and relevance to his or her own goals (potential advantage) before they engage in doping. This supports the notion that athletes who dope do it to satisfy a need (high performance or winning) and not to harm an opponent or break a rule (defiance) as has been the basis for most anti-doping campaigns (e.g. play clean! or just say no!) (Backhouse et al., 2015). Therefore, it seems prudent that baseline research seeking to understand the doping problem digs into meanings that people attach to doping and the needs they aim to solve. Once all these are done, only then can a discussion on healthier (safer, easier, or cheaper) alternatives be initiated.

Table 9.1 also presents perceptions on the likelihood of undesirable consequences (e.g. ability to self-regulate) and the role of pertinent environmental factors as other important schema elements. Athletes are often aware of the desirable effects of PES use. However, information about the harmful effects of doping behaviour may be deficient. This highlights the importance of including some deterrent components in anti-doping educational programmes even though the primary goal of anti-doping education is doping prevention. As such, educational programmes that are based on the systemic model need to highlight roles of existing testing institutions and consequences of a positive testing result on personnel and career.

The Role of Environmental and Personal Factors

The systemic model emphasises the importance of the interaction between a person and his or her environment in shaping doping decisions. Johnson (2012) contends that a person makes decisions which contribute to and are influenced by that person's environmental feedback. In his conceptualisation of this relationship, a triangle representing a person was placed as the fulcrum that found itself between environmental pressures and doping behaviour on a triple-beam balance. Through this he demonstrated how the relative weight of environmental factors such as the presence of an authority figure (motivational climate, Table 9.1) or the shift in the position of the triangle (personal feelings, thoughts, and behaviours – which may be affected by brain development or age) over time has a bearing on whether doping occurs. Moreover, the shift in the person alone mediates the amount of pressure the environment must impose for doping to occur. Factoring the role of this interplay in the design of baseline research or development of anti-doping programmes, considerations must be made at the level of the athlete as well as his or her immediate environment which includes his or her social climate, cultural norms, and athlete support personnel (Table 9.1).

9.5 Conclusion

Malawi faces a challenge in implementing the preventative and enforcement functions of the world anti-doping programme. This is manifested by the lack of comprehensive and evidence-based programmes on the ground. The problem is multifactorial. However, the front and centre of this problem are scarcity of prevalence data, limited understanding of the role of contextual factors in doping, and the absence of strong enforcement institutions. These contribute to limit adaptability of international standards to local contexts and frustrate potential development of anti-doping programmes. This chapter has appealed that action research based on the wide-spanning systemic model of doping behaviour can sufficiently inform design and implementation of a culturally responsive anti-doping educational programme in Malawi. This serves to inform future research and interventions for Malawi and other southern African nations.

References

Al Ghobain, M., Konbaz, M. S., Almassad, A., Alsultan, A., Al Shubaili, M., & AlShabanh, O. (2016). 'Prevalence, Knowledge, and Attitude of Prohibited Substances Use (Doping) Among Saudi Sport Players.' *Substance Abuse: Treatment, Prevention, and Policy, 11*(1), 1–6. https://doi.org/10.1186/s13011-016-0058-1

Aljaloud, S. O., Khoshhal, K. I., Al-Ghaiheb, A. A., Konbaz, M. S., & Almasaed, A. A. (2020). 'The Prevalence of Doping Among Saudi Athletes: Results from the National Anti-Doping Program.' *Journal of Taibah University Medical Sciences, 15*(1), 19–24. https://doi.org/10.1016/j.jtumed.2019.12.001

Backhouse, S., Whitaker, L., Patterson, L., Erickson, K., & Mckenna, J. (2015). *Social Psychology of Doping in Sport: A Mixed-Studies Narrative Synthesis.* Project report. World Anti-Doping Agency, Montreal Canada. 2016.

Bahrke, M., & Yasalis, C. (2002). 'History of Doping in Sports.' *International Sports Studies, 24*(1), 2002.

Bartlett, F. (1932). *Remembering: A Study in Experimental and Social Psychology.* Cambridge University Press.

Bird, S. R., Goebel, C., Burke, L. M., & Greaves, R. F. (2016). 'Doping in Sport and Exercise: Anabolic, Ergogenic, Health and Clinical Issues.' *Annals of Clinical Biochemistry, 53*(2), 196–221. https://doi.org/10.1177/0004563215609952

Brewer, W., & Nakamura, G. (1984). 'The Nature and Functions of Schemas.' In R. S. Wyer, Jr. & T. K. Srull (Eds.) *University of Illinois at Urbana-Champaign* (Vol. 13). University of Illinois.

Bronfenbrenner, U. (1977). 'Toward an Experimental Ecology of Human Development.' *American Psychologist, 32*(7), 513.

Bronfenbrenner, U. (1979). *The Ecology of Human Development: Experiments by Nature and Design*. Harvard University Press.

Bronfenbrenner, U. (2001). `Bioecological Theory of Human Development.' In N. J. Smelser & P. B. Baltes (Eds.), *International Encyclopaedia of the Social and Behavioural Sciences* (pp. 6963–6970). Elsevier.

Canadian Centre for Ethics in Sports. (2022). *World Anti-Doping Programme*. CCES. https://cces.ca/world-anti-doping-program

Chebet, S. (2014). *Evaluation of Knowledge, Attitudes, and Practices of Doping Among Elite Middle- and Long-Distance Runners in Kenya: A thesis*. Kenyatta University Institutional Repository, November.

Chinoko, C. (July 2, 2016). *Anti-Doping Body to Intensify Awareness*. The Nation Online. www.mwnation.com

Chisati, E. M., Undi, D., Ulili, S., Nkhoma, S., & Mlongoti, M. (2022). 'Prevalence of Performance Enhancing Substance Use Among Elite Football Players in Two Super League Teams in Blantyre, Malawi.' *Malawi Medical Journal, 34*(3), 157–161. https://doi.org/10.4314%2Fmmj.v34i3.3

Connor, J. M., & Mazanov, J. (2009). 'Would You Dope? A General Population Test of the Goldman Dilemma.' *British Journal of Sports Medicine, 43*(11), 871–872. https://doi.org/10.1136/bjsm.2009.057596

de Hon, O., Kuipers, H., & van Bottenburg, M. (2014). 'Prevalence of Doping Use in Elite Sports: A Review of Numbers and Methods.' *Sports Medicine, 45*(1), 57–69. https://doi.org/10.1007/s40279-014-0247-x

Dorota, S. E., & Derman, W. (2016). 'Anti-Doping Knowledge and Opinions of South African Pharmacists and General Practitioners.' *Journal of Sports Medicine & Doping Studies*, 6(3). https://doi.org/10.4172/2161-0673.1000181

European Commission. (2014). *Study on Doping Prevention: A Map of Legal, Regulatory and Prevention Practice Provisions in EU (European Union) 28*. European Commission. https://doi.org/10.2766/86776

Faiss, R., Saugy, J., Zollinger, A., Robinson, N., Schuetz, F., Saugy, M., & Garnier, P. Y. (2020). 'Prevalence Estimate of Blood Doping in Elite Track and Field Athletes During Two Major International Events.' *Frontiers in Physiology, 11*(February), 1–11. https://doi.org/10.3389/fphys.2020.00160

Gatterer, K., Gumpenberger, M., Overbye, M., Streicher, B., Schobersberger, W., & Blank, C. (2020). 'An Evaluation of Prevention Initiatives by 53 National Anti-Doping Organizations: Achievements and Limitations'. *Journal of Sport and Health Science, 9*(3), 228–239. https://doi.org/10.1016/j.jshs.2019.12.002

Gibbons, F. X., Gerrard, M., Blanton, H., & Russell, D. W. (1998). 'Reasoned Action and Social Reaction: Willingness and Intention as Independent Predictors of Health

Risk.' *Journal of Personality and Social Psychology, 74*(5), 1164–1180. https://doi.org/10.1037/0022-3514.74.5.1164

Gradidge, P., Coopoo, Y., & Constantinou, D. (2011). 'Prevalence of Performance-Enhancing Substance Use by Johannesburg Male Adolescents Involved in Competitive High School Sports.' *Archives of Exercise in Health and Disease, 2*(2), 114–119. https://doi.org/10.5628/aehd.v2i2.102

Johnson, M. B. (2011). 'A Systemic Model of Doping Behaviour.' *American Journal of Psychology, 124*(2), 151–162. https://doi.org/10.5406/amerjpsyc.124.2.0151

Johnson, M. B. (2012). 'A Systemic Social-Cognitive Perspective on Doping.' *Psychology of Sport and Exercise, 13*(3), 317–323. https://doi.org/10.1016/j.psychsport.2011.12.007

Kabiri, S., Willits, D. W., & Shadmanfaat, S. M. (2019). 'A Multi-Theoretical Framework for Assessing Performance-Enhancing Drug Use: Examining the Utility of Self-Control, Social Learning, and Control Balance Theories.' *Journal of Drug Issues, 49*(3), 512–530. https://doi.org/10.1177/0022042619839935

Kaoche, J. M. (2019). *Evaluation of Knowledge and Attitude on Doping by Football Athletes, Coaches and Sponsors in Malawi (Thesis) (Vol. 01, Issue 01)*. Kenyatta University.

Kaoche, J. M. C., Rintaugu, E. G., Kamenju, J., & Mwangi, F. M. (2020). 'Knowledge on Doping Among Football Athletes, Coaches and Sponsors in Malawi.' *Journal of Physical Education and Sport Management, 11*(December), 5–13. https://doi.org/10.5897/JPESM2020.0346

Morente-Sánchez, J., & Zabala, M. (2013). 'Doping in Sport: A Review of Elite Athletes' Attitudes, Beliefs, and Knowledge.' *Sports Medicine, 43*(6), 395–411. https://doi.org/10.1007/s40279-013-0037-x

Muwonge, H., Zavuga, R., & Kabenge, P. A. (2015). 'Doping Knowledge, Attitudes, and Practices of Ugandan Athletes: A Cross-Sectional Study.' *Substance Abuse: Treatment, Prevention, and Policy, 10*(1), 1–9. https://doi.org/10.1186/s13011-015-0033-2

Nyasatimes. (2013, September). *Malawi Intensifies Battle Against Doping in Sport: UNESCO Trains 30 Sport Managers*. Nyasa Times Malawi. https://www.nyasatimes.com

Ogden, J. (2015). 'Time to Retire the Theory of Planned Behaviour? One of Us Will Have to Go! A Commentary on Sniehotta, Presseau and Araújo-Soares.' *Health Psychology Review, 9*(2), 165–167. https://doi.org/10.1080/17437199.2014.898679

Sagoe, D., Molde, H., Andreassen, C. S., Torsheim, T., & Pallesen, S. (2014). 'The Global Epidemiology of Anabolic-Androgenic Steroid Use: A Meta-Analysis and Meta-Regression Analysis.' *Annals of Epidemiology, 24*(5), 383–398. https://doi.org/10.1016/j.annepidem.2014.01.009

Sagoe, D., Torsheim, T., Molde, H., Andreassen, C. S., & Pallesen, S. (2015). 'Attitudes Towards Use of Anabolic-Androgenic Steroids Among Ghanaian High School Students.' *International Journal of Drug Policy, 26*(2), 169–174. https://doi.org/10.1016/j.drugpo.2014.10.004

Shibata, K., Ichikawa, K., & Kurata, N. (2017). 'Knowledge of Pharmacy Students About Doping, and the Need for Doping Education: A Questionnaire Survey.' *BMC Research Notes, 10*(1), 396. https://doi.org/10.1186/s13104-017-2713-7

Sniehotta, F. F., Presseau, J., & Araújo-Soares, V. (2014). 'Time to Retire the Theory of Planned Behaviour.' *Health Psychology Review, 8*(1), 1–7. https://doi.org/10.1080/17437199.2013.869710

Whitaker, L., Backhouse, S. H., & Long, J. (2014). 'Reporting Doping in Sport: National Level Athletes' Perceptions of Their Role in Doping Prevention.' *Scandinavian Journal of Medicine and Science in Sports, 24*(6), e515–e521. https://doi.org/10.1111/sms.12222

Woolway, T., Lazuras, L., Barkoukis, V., & Petróczi, A. (2020). 'Doing What Is Right and Doing It Right: A Mapping Review of Athletes' Perception of Anti-Doping Legitimacy.' *International Journal of Drug Policy, 84*, 102865. https://doi.org/10.1016/j.drugpo.2020.102865

World Anti-doping Agency. (2021). *World Anti-Doping Code*. www.wada-ama.org

Chapter 10

"Witchcraft Doping" and Grassroots Sport Development

Frank George Mgungwe

10.1 Introduction

Posner (2008) advises that "sports are designed to highlight, isolate and display natural hierarchies of innate traits of man...such as height, strength, agility, beauty, physical coordination and brilliance" (p. 1729). However, some athletes use performance-enhancing substances and methods to outcompete their opponents (Morente-Sánchez & Zabala, 2013). This is commonly known as doping and is a complex problem in sports today prohibited worldwide (Obasa & Borry, 2019). The anti-doping monitoring and surveillance rests in the hands of the World Anti-Doping Agency (WADA, 2021). According to the WADA Code (2021), "anti-doping programs are founded on the intrinsic value of sport in how we play true" (p. 13).

WADA was created to promote, coordinate, and monitor the fight against using performance-enhancing substances in sports (Pugh & Pugh, 2019). However, as Kovac (2018) posits, strategies for anti-doping by WADA to curb and end doping are based on the separation of the body and the mind, the biological and the psychological, the physical and the spiritual. Kovac (2018) further notes that WADA prioritises the physical (not spiritual), where a clean athlete means being free from prohibited substances and methods. A lengthy list of chemicals deemed performance-enhancing substances and methods are banned (WADA, 2021). Still, methods and substances under witchcraft are missing even though Pannenborg (2010) advises to "be aware that juju is a serious affair and that most players and supporters strongly believe in it as it works on a psychological level and as such has a function in football" (p. 35) and, therefore, should never be ignored.

Traditional witchcraft sports medicine (*Juju*) is used in competitions such as football (Leseth, 2010). The contents of this chapter derive from phenomenological anecdotes. The data was generated over a lengthy period of four years (2018 to 2022) by recording observations of events unfolding before, during, and after the sporting event he attended. Out of interest, he recorded critical information in his "reflective journal" during these events with a vision to put them together for a future book on rural sports events or contribute to a

DOI: 10.4324/9781003370796-12

chapter like the current one. The author uses vignettes in the form of spoken narratives. The goal underpinning this decision is that narratives are likely to make the reader listen to key informants' stories, prioritising their voices and hearing their versions of experiences (Pring, 2004). He uses the terms "rural football" and "rural netball" to mean competitions initiated by Members of Parliament (MPs) or "shadow MPs" or significant others of the society, as opposed to official leagues run by the Football Association of Malawi (FAM) and Central Region Football League (CRFL) officials as authorities.

These rural football and netball competitions by MPs are not regularly commissioned like the mainstream official leagues. They are initiated at the convenience of MPs or when needed. For example, a year can pass without commissioning one, especially after an election year. But sometimes, twice or more cycles of competitions per year can be conducted as time gravitates towards general elections. The competitions can often be in leagues, bonanzas, and tournaments.

10.2 Literature on Witchcraft and Doping

Practices of witchcraft in Africa are real and are part of everyday reality (Wyk, 2004). In witchcraft belief system everything beyond common sense is attached to supernatural beliefs (Tebbe, 2007). Asamoah-Gyadu (2015) describes this as "African electronics" (p. 1). In Africa the existence of ghosts and witches is as real as the existence of electricity or magnetism (Welbourn, 1968, as quoted by Masanja, 2015). Also, Schmidt (2005) explains that "supernatural powers are real to Africans as electricity is real" (p. 17), since both cannot be seen but their effects in life are felt. In Africa, well learned, peasant farmers, Christians, and Muslims all believe in witchcraft existence (Wyk, 2004). Thus, Nyamnjoh (2017) notes that "words, deeds and beings are always incomplete, not because of absences but because of their possibilities" (p. 256).

According to Gram (2011), witchcraft is believed to disobey laws of nature and is highly capable of achieving the impossible. Muhanika (2011) claims that there is no evidence for proving or disapproving how witchcraft operates, for the whole business is an attitude of mind, camouflaged in secrecy, and reflects idealism at its worst. Thus, Pannenborg (2010) observes that opposing teams and their supporters "tend to see everybody as spies; people who are trying to find out their juju" (p. 33). According to Mafico (1986) in Wyk (2004), this explains why witchcraft has been studied by many social researchers for long, but the conclusions are as diverse as their number. Indeed, as Pannenborg (2010, p. 33) maintains, "If a team discovers the kind of juju of opposing team, they counter attack by neutralising it, and thus stakeholders keep the information to themselves".

In African societies, most people believe that activities of the living are controlled by unseen supernatural forces of other spirit world (Bryceson,

2010; Makulilo, 2010). Thus, most of the population rely on "traditional medicine" for many activities including primary health care and many other competitions, including sport (WHO, 2008). According to WHO (2008), traditional medicine is defined as all the skills, knowledge, and spiritual practices which are based on the theories, belief systems, and experiences endemic to different cultures that are used to detect, prevent, improve, or treat illnesses. Also, Richter (2003) elucidates that traditional medicine is a kind of personalised health care that is culturally appropriate, holistic, and tailored to meet the needs and expectations of the patient. Traditional medicine practitioners in Africa leverage on their connection to the supernatural powers in order to invoke fortune for those seeking help from them (Winkler et al., 2010). Lewis (2012) asserts that the health of African people everywhere has always depended on the holistic aspect of mind, body, and spirit.

Pannenborg (2010) observes that "much of the violence in African football is juju-related" (p. 35). Masanja (2015) quoting Welbourn (1968) asserts that in communities where witchcraft beliefs are strong, poverty, starvation, and illiteracy are predominant characteristics. Thus, in these communities, when misfortune hits a member or a family, witchcraft becomes a primary suspicion especially if natural explanations do not satisfy, compelling them to seek help from witch doctors to give explanations (Gufler, 1999). It is, therefore, obvious that witchcraft beliefs slow down social progress (Essien & Ben, 2011).

According to Chenya (1988), witch doctors are doctors who diagnose and heal sickness of the body and soul. They know medicinal trees, roots, and leaves from which medicines are produced. It is through dreams at night when they are commonly shown secret things by ancestors (Ouma, 2013). Indigenous knowledge is clear that witchcraft has been a common explanation for diseases of which the causes were unknown (The Voice, 2012). Witch doctors discover spiritual root causes of issues by navigating the supernatural causes (Mumo, 2012). According to Mbiti (1969) cited by Mumo (2012), in African view, health includes many aspects such as diseases, witchcraft, sorcery, curses, and misfortunes, which need attention from specialised practitioners to deal with.

Historically, it is believed that African traditional leaders (chiefs) relied on divination and mysticism (Mutiba, 2012). Magic is as vital as the training, and the witch doctor is as vital as the coach (Stollznow, 2010). It is no wonder that players would rather undergo spiritual rituals than to train hard to improve their football skills (Pannenborg, 2010). According to Botchway (2011), Africans believe in the existence and influence of unseen spirits and deities: the majority of the people consider it foolhardy to engage in a business venture or a social activity without first soliciting divine inspiration and intervention. According to Royer (2005), sports teams employ magicians for the belief that they can produce victory by either causing opposing team members to suffer blurred vision or causing the opponent's ball to slow down in mid-air. Thus, losing sports teams blame their loss on witchcraft, for it is well known that witch doctors are hired to help thwart the opposing team and thereby ensure victory.

However, Pannenborg (2010) explains that *Juju* is considered an African secret since players, coaches, and officials commonly deny that they are into *Juju* and claim to be Christians or Muslims and only pray when in fact the majority of football teams are in one way or the other involved in these spiritual practices. Those who believe in witchcraft are deeply convinced that practitioners in this field possess natural super powers (Muhanika, 2011). But according to Stolloznow (2010), whatever the activity may be, there is no alternative to proper planning, hard work, and professionalism.

The World Anti-Doping Code (WADC) is the fundamental document upon which this unified fight against doping is based (Obasa & Borry, 2019). According to Posner (2008), the challenge for sports doping is that it "has only a minor public dimension; its solution can largely be left to the free market" (p. 1743). He further notes that in sport "the choice to punish or promote doping does not have any great public significance" (p. 1735). WADA considers doping as fundamentally contrary to the spirit of sport (Pugh & Pugh, 2019). But WADA Code encourages national anti-doping organisations (NADOs) to support anti-doping research (WADA Code, 2021).

The term "doping" has been defined by WADA as the use of prohibited substances and methods designed to enhance performance in sport competitions (Obasa & Borry, 2019). However, Sandel (2007) considers doping as "the use of substances and technologies that improve and corrupt athletic competition as a human activity that honours the cultivation and display of natural talents" (p. 111). For Posner (2008), doping is "the use of substances and technologies that disturb or obscure the natural talent that sports seek to exhibit" (p. 1731). WADA has given a list of substances which it calls prohibited list for any use by those partaking in competitions (for full prohibited list, see WADA, 2022). Some drugs are banned both in and out of competition due to their performance-enhancing properties, while others are only banned during competition (Read et al., 2019). The primary focus in curbing doping has been on testing athletes and the development of tests to detect their usage (Morente-Sánchez & Zabala, 2013).

Unlike in societies outside Africa, the other form of performance-enhancing substances or methods in sports in rural Africa uses "witchcraft doping" where sport competitors or teams outsource the services of a shaman or magician or sorcerer, or warlock, or herbalists or commonly witch doctor. In African societies, the terms "traditional healers", "witch doctors", or "herbalists" in principle are the same thing and therefore in most cases the words are used interchangeably (Beck, 1979). The terms "witchcraft doping" and "spiritual doping" are used interchangeably to mean the same thing: covert use of performance-enhancing substances and/or methods thought to carry supernatural powers to influence sport competition outcome. Sport medicine is commonly known as *Juju* and the generic name for actual mystical object used is *Chinthumwa*.

Globally, the largest anti-doping organisation is WADA, which has so far developed a coordinated, worldwide anti-doping programme that applies to sports that have signed a pledge to uphold the WADA Code (Pugh & Pugh, 2019). The WADA Code outlines their anti-doping policies, rules, and regulations with sport organisations and amongst public authorities around the world. More than 660 sports organisations have signed the WADA Code including the International Olympic and Paralympic Committees, all Olympic Sport International Federations, and National Olympic and Paralympic Committees. The practical application of the WADA regulations is performed by national anti-doping agencies. Malawi Anti-Doping Organisation (MADO) was formed and became operational in 2013.

How is a substance included? What does it take for a substance to be included in the WADA Prohibited List? According to the WADA Code (2021, p. 32), a substance or method will be considered for the WADA Prohibited List if the substance or method meets any two of the following three criteria:

a It has the potential to enhance or enhances sport performance.
b It represents an actual or potential health risk to the athlete.
c It violates the spirit of sport.

10.3 Methodology

As Onyinah (2015) puts it, "witchcraft is considered spiritual, complex and very secret that cannot be monitored or evaluated by scientific methods" (p. 1). In this regard, Luyaluka (2017) quoting N'sakila (1986) observes that abstractive induction is a better methodology of studying witchcraft for it is considered "a social reality whose existence is judged by its effects on the physical plane and by its diverse expressions in social life" (p. 633). Thus, data about "witchcraft doping" in football can better be extracted principally by analysing rumours and accusations and filtering truths. The contents of this chapter derive from phenomenological anecdotes of the author. The data was generated over a period of four years (2018 to 2022) through observations of events before, during, and after the sport event the researcher watched. These were supported by narratives from rural sport administrators, coaches supporters, and players. Out of interest, he was recording key information in his reflective journal during these events. Also, data was collected through one-on-one interview with five traditional sports medicine practitioners.

Ethical Considerations

The researcher is fully cognisant of basic common law obligations that obligation of confidence arises spontaneously when one generates or is in possession of information he knows is very secret by the type of information in question. Therefore, a breach of confidence will arise if the researcher misuses and abuses this information. The inherent rights to privacy of interviewees should therefore not be violated in any way. Thus, against this backdrop, every interviewee took part consensually.

10.4 How Does "Witchcraft Doping" in Rural Football Occur?

Pannenborg (2010) observes that

> there are different forms of juju in football…for instance the head of a cat, a needle and a piece of paper with names of the opponent team players may be buried on the pitch or near the entrance to the stadium.
>
> (p. 33)

Since the tradition of knowledge in Africa is informed by and relate to all domains of life and the environment (Nel, 2008), it follows that in traditional sport medicine, resources mostly in use include small pieces of particular herbs (root, leaves, stems, and barks), tree bark pieces or threads, animal skin, liver, gall bladder, and/or any animal tissue. But mostly, all these are made to a general end-user product commonly called *Chinthumwa*, a final product carrying all the designated spiritual forces. Also, talismans can be made and worn on the wrist, in the waist, and/or as a necklace. To conceal these and avoid being caught, end users hide them in their boots, or in the rubber band sockets of their shorts. Some preparations can be in the form of herb potions prepared for end users to drink, and wash their feet, hands, or body.

Indeed, Pannenborg (2010) claims that "spirits too may appear on the pitch to disrupt play" (p. 33). It is noted that witch doctors draw their winning power from their special relationships with the spiritual ancestors (Tebbe, 2007). According to Asamoah-Gyadu (2015), "witchcraft is a neutral supernatural power that may be used either for good or for ill" (p. 1). Onyinah (2015) similarly notes that "the distinctive characteristic of harming by witchcraft is that it is done in secret; it is the imperceptible projection of inducement from the witch to the target victim" (p. 1). Further, Onyinah (2015) claims that "witches can frustrate the good plans of people…through spiritual manipulations" (p. 1). Pannenborg (2010) contends that "juju brings luck to one team and bad luck to the other" (p. 33). Thus, in sport, witchcraft can be used to substantively and momentarily incapacitate opponents during game time or prevent opponents from scoring by creating an invisible repulsive force to any ball shooting.

Indigenous knowledge hands down to each generation that witchcraft attacks are most likely to occur in such competitions to incapacitate the opponent, and therefore, one needs self-protection for better participation. Enrolling into a sport competition without being spiritually doped is considered a clear own risk and very dangerous. Luyaluka (2017) quoting N'sakila (1986) observes that witchcraft "is judged by its effects on the physical plane and by its diverse expressions in social life" (p. 633).

Sport performance-enhancing methods are varied (Morente-Sánchez & Zabala, 2013), and those through witchcraft practices are eclectic in both their sources and their intended line of action to influence the desired result of a sports game. A wide range of resource substances and materials are used, including parts of particular trees such as leaves, barks, and roots, parts of animal tissues or organs such as intestines, testes, and horns, and human tissues such as hair. In terms of line of action and use, these witchcraft resources are mixed in proportions which work in same wavelength with incantation spells to function at least within the dimensions of the match or competition in question. The resultant occult powers, though durational, can produce highly effective spiritual repulsive-force for any ball-shooting targeted on goal posts, especially by opponents. Society believes that this is the hidden, unseen cause of extraordinarily unusual misfiring and misses by opponents during highly competed football and netball matches. Let us now navigate through the following vignettes which are synthesised from the games watched by the author.

10.5 Instances Which Reflect Convincingly Effective "Witchcraft Doping"

As already seen above, in rural football, rumours, speculations, and accusations of "witchcraft doping" characterise match build-up conversations, the atmosphere of which gets fierce as the game starts and progresses. Asamoah-Gyadu (2015) describes witchcraft as African electronics (p. 1). The *Chinthumwa* used in sports is the "electronic gadget", equipment specially made to work according to the wishes of the stakeholder. Using vignettes, let us go through the events.

Vignette 1

After the game between Team K and Team R in a constituency league, a conflict ensued amongst players of the same team: "I told you guys that we need to follow instructions of the witchdoctor that we should not sleep at our homes. Look now, we have lost! Surely, someone here slept with his wife that's why we have lost this game. We should have slept at one place to avoid this", rued one player to the loss. Avoiding sleeping with anyone was one of the key conditions of the outsourced sport medicine.

Vignette 2

In a certain constituency league game: "Guys, let's not go to the dressing room. They have 'contaminated' it with charm potions to incapacitate us", charges the coach in Chichewa at halftime. Supporters echoing, "Let's just be here!" He adds as he moves into the pitch. Then one man, camouflaging as a supporter, but a "consulted wizard" performs some invocations and cryptic doings. He then points a mystical object at his team's goal to cast repulsive forces at it, so no shooting is targeted". This team won the match by two goals to nil.

Vignette 3

There were heavy accusations of "witchcraft doping" before the match between Team X and Team Y. Team X accused Team Y of contaminating the pitch with potions. Also, Team Y accused Team X of contaminating the pitch with potions. The match was scheduled to commence at 14:30 hrs and the referee blew his whistle many times in wait but players could not appear near the pitch. Each one waited for the other team to start stepping on the pitch. Long at last after queries from people who patronised to watch the game, Team Y started stepping on the Pitch. They entered the pitch through the corner. Then Team X also entered the pitch through the same corner. Team Y, which started entering the pitch lost the game by three goals to one. It was conclusive that the sport medicine for the first team to enter the pitch was neutralised by the second team, and so the medicine of the second team worked.

Vignette 4

Rumour of "witchcraft doping" was rife in the build-up conversations amongst supporters before the match between Team P and Team Q. Each team accused the other of "witchcraft doping". These were Quarter Finals. The game ended in a one-all draw. During extra time recess, all the four strikers of Team Q removed their jerseys and wore them inside out. They also applied pork fat on their boots. Within the remaining minutes, two of these strikers scored the winning goals. In this match, the power of *Juju* for both teams appeared to have matched and to have operated equally at the same wavelength, and hence the draw in the first ninety minutes. The changing of jerseys to inside out by strikers of Team Q and the application of pork fat on their boots neutralised and obscured the *Juju* pattern of the opposing team which ultimately guaranteed the win.

Vignette 5

In a certain constituency netball league, the build-up conversations to a netball game between Team G and Team H were characterised by accusations of "witchcraft doping". Team G players accused players of Team H to have spiritually doped the match ball and they refused to allow it in. Likewise, Team H players accused players of Team G to have spiritually doped their ball and they refused to allow it in. The game was scheduled to commence at 15:00 hrs but due to the squabbles, it began at 15:43 hrs after officials brought in a neutral ball. The game ended eleven baskets apiece.

Vignette 6

In a certain constituency netball league, the build-up conversations to a netball game between Team C and Team D were characterised by accusations of "witchcraft doping". The game started at 14:30 hrs normally, but before the end of first quarter, two players of Team D complained of extreme tiredness and feeling too heavy to continue playing, accusing their opponents to have caused this. "My legs are too heavy to effectively run when in the court of play, but relieved when am out. They have bewitched us", charged one girl as she exited the court. This Team D lost by 17 baskets to 23 baskets.

Vignette 7

Amongst supporters of both teams, rumour speculation of "witchcraft doping" was highly rife in the build-up conversations before the match between Team M, the minnows and Team N, the favourites. Each team accused their opponents of "witchcraft doping". Before the commencement of the match, the pitch was searched heavily by match officials. Pig fat and salt with some semi-solid potions were found tied using a dark tree-bark rope. This game was characterised by numerous unusual misfiring and misses by both teams beyond natural comprehension. The game ended in a goalless draw. In the second half of extra time in the thick of the game, the referee blew the whistle for a foul, far away from the goal posts, but to the amazement of everyone, one striker of Team N, solely moved the ball towards the goal of the opposite team "until he scored", aimed just to pass the ball and himself on the goal line. Everyone was shocked! This act was meant to neutralise or quell the repulsive force claimed to have hovered around the goal posts by "witchcraft doping" which was responsible for the unusual misses and misfiring of his team during the first ninety minutes of the game. The player was shown a yellow card for this misconduct. Within three minutes the striker scored and they won the game by one goal to zero.

As can be noted in these vignettes, the attempted doping convincingly reflects effectiveness of "witchcraft doping" because the teams which doped emerged victors and thus it is conclusive that "witchcraft doping" had helped the teams secure their victories.

10.6 Instances Which Reflect Clear Failure of Attempted "Witchcraft Doping"

Vignette 1

After the game between Team D, the favourites, and Team E, the underdogs, in a constituency league, a verbal conflict ensued amongst players of the latter: "He is fake, very stupid. How can we lose to these children? Where is he?" the captain angrily charges in Chichewa as he jostles out of the pitch. The consulted wizard had left some minutes earlier, fearing reproach. This Team E had followed all the "witchcraft doping" instructions given to them by the consulted wizard.

Vignette 2

In a match between Team A and Team B for a constituency league, Team A outsourced the traditional witchcraft sport medicine from a particular seasoned sport medicine practitioner within the same community. But contrary to the expectations of every stakeholder of the team on the day of the match, the first-choice goalkeeper refused to follow instructions of wearing a talisman in his waist, like all other players: "No, I can't have that on my body. For what? If it means a loss, let it be". The team failed to have him out of the first eleven. He played. This goalkeeper made amazingly great saves and unanimously in the eyes of all who watched the game, he was the Man of the Match. They won by four goals to two.

Vignette 3

Constituency League: In the build-up conversations before the match between Team K and Team L, rumour speculation of "witchcraft doping" was highly rife, the latter accused the former of "witchcraft doping". On the eve of the match, Team K camped at one place to ensure that all instructions of "witchcraft doping" were followed. All players complied with the instructions. The first team to get into the pitch was Team L. When entering the pitch, all players of Team K used one corner and ran around the pitch in a "warm up" exercise, and had worn a talisman on their wrists. Team L won this game by five goals to two. At the end of the match, one player rued: "this doping has betrayed, it's very fake, complete fake...we should have just concentrated on our game plan!"

Vignette 4

In a Constituency League game between Sechaba (pseudonym) FC and Kokeni (pseudonym) FC, there was a fierce fight and violence amongst supporters. These were semi-finals and the referee and other officials were imported from Lilongwe. The game was scheduled to kick off at 14:00 hrs but it was delayed until 15:00 hrs. Each team waited for the opponents to start entering the pitch. It took the intervention of officials from the sponsor that Sechaba FC started entering the pitch. Then players of Kokeni FC entered the pitch using a minibus (and with their outsourced man to serve them with sport medicine), which drove round the opponents three times (presumably to unscrew the sport medicine of opponents and make theirs lively intact). Then one man alighted from the minibus and started shouting in a mixture of Tonga and Chichewa: "yeah you are in for it today! We have sealed everything: we have tethered you! No chance!" But before the second half, Sechaba FC was leading by two goals to nil. In the second half when Sechaba FC scored a third goal about 12 minutes before full time, Kokeni FC supporters invaded the pitch and violence ensued. The referee and linesman were severely beaten by Kokeni FC supporters – "witchcraft doping" for Kokeni FC did not work.

In the multiplicity of being in African thought system, something can be and at the same time cannot be (Nyamnjoh, 2012). These instances demonstrate a clear failure of attempted "witchcraft doping", and the incompleteness of things advanced by Nyamnjoh (2017). In the first set of vignettes, "witchcraft doping" appears to create a false-positive illusion of effectiveness in competitors which influenced their on-the-pitch performance. In most competitions, especially those tournaments, bonanzas and leagues initiated by influential figures, such as Members of Parliaments (MPs) in their jurisdictions, rumour speculations, and accusations of spiritual doping characterise event build-up conversations. Each team and supporters strongly accuse their opponents of spiritual doping. Sometimes, this is also the case with inter-school Malawi Schools Sports Association (MASSA) games, whether friendly or competed for, in primary section and secondary schools, the two-tier feeder leagues for the regional leagues, Super League, and the national team.

10.7 How "Witchcraft Doping" Provides Challenges to Initiatives by WADA to Control Doping

Pannenborg (2010) notes that "children see the players of the big teams performing juju on the pitch and immediately want to copy what they are doing. That's why these beliefs will never cease to exist" (p. 34). Similarly, Schmidt (2005) claims that "it is a natural assumption for Africans that mystical powers interfere with our life" (p. 17). These strong beliefs in witchcraft breed suspicion, hatred, and jealousy amongst players. According to Pannenborg (2010), a big and long injury of a popular player causes him or her to think that his team mates on the dugout have bewitched him or her in order to secure his or her playing time. This is a clear issue retarding sport development.

To this far, doping has long been a matter of private concern for sport insiders until the late 1990s (Hoberman, 2001). Røkke (2004) argues that in the light of tradition of indigenous knowledge African witch doctors are considered as the link to the ancestors with the belief that the latter are more powerful and have influence on their living descendants. This makes witch doctors to be key characters in their respective communities. Therefore, spiritual assistance in such communities is important and revered in order for one to obtain good life on earth (Westlund, 2006). Wyk (2004, p. 43) posits that witchcraft has been one of the biggest challenges facing humanity, and that "Witchcraft is an expression of jealousy and hatred" (Pannenborg, 2010, p. 34).

According to Posner (2008), "sports are designed to highlight, isolate and display natural hierarchies of innate traits" of man such as "height, strength, agility, beauty, physical coordination and brilliance" (p. 1729). Sandel (2007) observes that doping is bad because it distorts and overrides these natural talents, making it difficult to measure progress. Thus, doping creates an unfair advantage over those athletes who refrain from doping and choose to participate without doping as expected, relying only on their own ability. In "witchcraft doping", players train minimally or "would rather undergo spiritual rituals than to train hard to improve their football skills" (Pannenborg, 2010, p. 34). Thus, although Stollznow (2010) asserts that witchcraft sport medicine is important like the training, and the witch doctor is also vital as the coach, the minimal training by players is a great covert hindrance to skill acquisition.

Posner (2008) notes that the major challenge of sports doping is that it has only a minor public dimension (more so "witchcraft doping" and its solution can largely be left to the free market). According to Pannenborg (2010), "juju is considered an African secret which is aimed at weakening the opponent team to give one's team more chances in winning the match" (p. 33). Should "witchcraft doping" in sport covertly prevalent in some rural Africa be left to the free market? For me, the correct answer is "no" if the fight against doping is to be effective, especially where superstitious beliefs are prevalent. Practices of witchcraft in sport competitions are highly esoteric and are thus a contentious issue when stakeholders in a competition in question have experienced it, believe in its powers, or do the practice themselves. Thus, although Pannenborg (2010) thinks "whatever else juju does, it fulfils an important psychological function" (p. 34), *Juju* is a retrogressive agent to sport development not only in Malawi, but across Africa as well.

10.8 Conclusion

Regularly watching football and netball competitions in rural communities in Malawi gives an excellent vantage lens to appreciate the extent to which witchcraft sport medicine becomes a bottleneck to the development of sport in the country. As can be noted in the vignettes, rumour and accusations on witchcraft in sports, particularly football and netball, retard skill nurturing and harnessing and, consequently, the general development of sports in Malawi. Engaging in "witchcraft doping" creates a false-positive illusion of effectiveness in competitors which affects or influences their substantive on-the-pitch performance like in placebo effect. This is so because when people start "witchcraft doping", they stop or reduce investing in their practices and physical efforts for upskilling and re-skilling, technically and tactically to highlight, isolate the natural hierarchies of innate traits (Posner, 2008). Therefore, any "witchcraft doping" in sport should never be permitted unless according to Posner (2008), "to the extent it improves a sport in the eyes of the spectators" (p. 1735). Thus, "witchcraft doping" can be seen as one form of multiplicities of being in African indigenous knowledge system and unless it gets admitted into WADA prohibited list, the anti-doping fight is a far-fetched dream especially in African countries (Nyamnjoh, 2012).

All stakeholders in sports should primarily understand the creed of the Olympics, which clearly states that "the important thing in the games is not winning but taking part and that the essential thing is not conquering, but fighting well" (Wheating, 2018, p. 1). The use of witchcraft sport medicine occurring deep in rural areas is an underlying bottleneck to sport development in Malawi, requiring authorities such as MADO officials, Malawi National Council of Sports (MNCS) officials, and FAM officials to effectively and continuously cascade down WADA Code to them. This is so because as team members continue concentrating on "witchcraft doping" by outsourcing witchcraft services, they stop or invest less in their practices and training for acquisition and improvement of skills both technically and tactically, believing that supernatural occult powers would enable them secure victory.

Positionality Statement

I have been a district vice chairperson for MASSA for three years and sports master in several rural secondary schools, and through these positions, I have made a great network and relationships with colleagues, players, rural football coaches, referees, and rural football and netball administrators. I want to acknowledge that this positionality within the ambits of this work and, therefore, my own lenses on the data generated through anecdotes of my reflective journal might have influenced or contributed positively or negatively to interpretations of the situations as they occurred before, during, and after the sport events. I picked the most interesting aspects of the unfolding events in my reflective journal. Since these were of interest to me, I might be ignoring other important aspects which would have helped me in interpreting the vignettes. Thus, I acknowledge that to some extent my positionality might influenced the writing exercise of this work and especially from personal interactions and experiences of rural football.

Acknowledgements

I thank the following officers for their invaluable commentaries and information in locating the right sources of information to enable me write and augment this piece of work: Mr. Chimwemwe Fedson (Chairperson for MASSA in Nkhotakota district), Mr. Patrick Chazama (Desk Officer for Sports for Kasungu district), Mr. I.O. Kakusa (Nkhotakota District Chairperson for Netball Association of Malawi – NAM), Mr. Herbert Chisusu (Sports Officer for Nkhotakota LEA Primary School), Mr. Blessings Marley (Sports Officer for Nkhotakota district), Mr. Samson Kalikokha Chimangeni (Malomo Community Day Secondary School), and Mr. P. Ching'ombe of Malomo Post Office and Mr. Sylvester Mwase (Malomo Community Day Secondary School). Most importantly, I thank Dr. Yamikani Ndauka and Dr. Simon Makwinja for accepting my chapter to be part of the book and their guidance and great support throughout the writing process.

References

Asamoah-Gyadu, K. (2015). *Witchcraft: Tension Between Protection and Destruction*. Retrieved from https://henrycenter.tiu.edu/2015/07/witchcraft-tension-between-protection-and-destruction/

Beck, A. (1979). Traditional Healer in Tanzania. *A Journal of Opinion, 9*(3): 2–5. Retrieved from www-jstor-org.nottingham.idm.oclc.org/stable/1166255?sid=primo&seq=1

Botchway, F. J. (2011). *Book Preview: Juju, Magic and Witchcraft in African Football*. Retrieved from: www.ghanaweb.com/GhanaHomePage/SportsArchive/artikel.php?ID=222635

Bryceson, D.F., Jonsson, J. B., & Sherrington, R. (2010). Miners' Magic: Artisnal Mining, the Albino Fetish and Murder. *Tanzania. Journal of Modern African Studies*. https://doi:10.1017/S0022278X10000303

Chenya, J. H. (1988). Imani za jadi za Kisukuma katika misemo, hadithi, Methali, na Desturi za Maisha. CID Edition. Tabora, Tanzania.

Essien, A., & Ben, V. (2011). New Paradigm in Witchcraft Issues: A Strategic Procedure for Sustainable Development in Nigeria. *American Journal of Social and Management Sciences, 2*(1): 47–55. https://doi.org/10.5251/ajsms.2011.2.1.47.55

Gram, D. (2011). *Child Witches and Witch Hunts: New Images of the Occult in the Democratic Republic of Congo*. Harvard Humanitarian Initiative.

Gufler, H. (1999). Witchcraft beliefs among the Yamba (Cameroon). *Anthropods, 94*: 181–198. Retrieved from: www.jstor.org/stable/40465701

Hoberman, J. (2001). *How Drug Testing Fails: The Politics of Doping Control in Doping in Elite Sport: The Politics of Drugs in the Olympic Movement*. World Athletics.

Kovac, U. (2018). Juju: Africa doping. *The Independent*. Retrieved from; www.independent.co.ug/juju-africa-doping/2/

Leseth, A. (2010). *Michezo: Dance, Sports and Politics in Tanzania*. Slovene Anthropological Society: Center for the Study of Professions. Retrieved from: www.researchgate.net/publication/265247003

Lewis, N. (2012). *What Is the African Traditional Herbal Research Clinic?* African Traditional Herbal Research Clinic Newsletter. Retrieved from http://docs.mak.ac.ug/sites/default/files/atcNewsletter412_0.pdf

Luyaluka, K. L. (2017). An Empirical Methodology of the Study of Witchcraft and Its Implementation in African Cultures. *Saudi Journal of Humanities and Social Sciences, 2*(8), 633–642. Retrieved from: https://DOI:10.21276/sjhss.

Makulilo, E. B. (2010). *Albino Killings in Tanzania: Witchcraft and Racism?* Retrieved from www.academia.edu/Documents/in/Albino_killings_and_media_coverage

Masanja, M. (2015). Albinos' Plight: Will Legal Methods be Powerful Enough to Eradicate Albinos' Scourge? *International Journal of Education and Research*. Retrieved from www.ijern.com/journal/2015/May-2015/20.pdf

Morente-Sánchez, J., & Zabala, M. (2013). Doping in Sport: A Review of Elite Athletes' Attitudes, Beliefs and Knowledge. *Sports Med*. Retrieved from http://dx.doi.org/10.1007/s40279-013-0037-x

Muhanika, H. (2011). *Why Controversy on Loliondo Magic Healer Is Inevitable*. Retrieved from www.ippmedia.com/frontend/index.php?l=27472

Mumo, P. M. (2012). Holistic Healing: An Analytical Review of Medicine-men in African Societies. *Thought and Practice: A Journal of the Philosophical Association of Kenya, 4*(1): 111–122. Retrieved from: https://philpapers.org/asearch.pl?pub=4633

Mutiba, B. G. (2012). A Cultural Approach to Development, Governance, and Democracy in Africa. Retrieved from: https://bagumageraldmutiba.wordpress.com/2012/03/03/a-cultural-approach-todevelopment-governance-and-democracy-in-africa-baguma-gerald-mutiba/

Nel, P. (2008). *Indigenous Knowledge in Africa: Challenges and Opportunities*. Centre for Africa Studies. Retrieved from: www.ufs.ac.za/docs/librariesprovider20/centre-for-africa-studies-documents/all-documents/osman-lecture-1788-eng.pdf?sfvrsn.

Nyamnjoh, F. B. (2012). Blinded by Sight: Divining the Future of Anthropology in Africa. *Africa Spectrum, 47*(3). Retrieved from: www.jstor.org/stable/23350451

Nyamnjoh, F. B. (2017). Incompleteness: Frontier Africa and the Currency of Conviviality. *Journal of Tropical Futures, 52*(3). Retrieved from: https://doi.org/10.1177/0021909615580867

Obasa, M., & Borry, P. (2019). The Landscape of the "Spirit of Sport": A Systematic Review. *Journal of Bioethical Inquiry, 16*: 443–453. Retrieved from https://doi.org/10.1007/s11673-019-09934-0

Onyinah, O. (2015). *The Activities of Witches. Church and Culture*. Retrieved from https://henrycenter.tiu.edu/2015/06/the-activities-of-witches/

Ouma, K. (2013). Fighting Witch. Retrieved from: https://dengeki.fandom.com/wiki/Fighting_Witch

Pannenborg, A. (2010). *Football in Africa: Observations about Political, Financial, Cultural and Religious Influences*. Sports and Dev.

Posner, R. A. (2008). In Defense of Prometheus: Some Ethical, Economic, and Regulatory Issues of Sports Doping. *Duke Law Journal*. Retrieved from: www.jstor.org/stable/40040631

Pring, R. (2004). *Philosophy of Educational Research* (2nd ed.). London: Continuum.

Pugh, J., & Pugh, C. (2019). Neurostimulation, Doping, and the Spirit of Sport. Retrieved from https://doi.org/10.1007/s12152-020-09435-7

Read, D., Skinner, J., Lock, D., & Houlihan, B. (2019). Legitimacy Driven Change at the World Anti-Doping Agency. *International Journal of Sport Policy and Politics, 11*(2), 233–245. Retrieved from https://doi.org/10.1080/19406940.2018.1544580

Richter, M. (2003) Traditional Medicines and Traditional Healers in South Africa. Discussion paper prepared for the Treatment Action Campaign and AIDS Law Project. AIDS Law Project. Retrieved from: www.counsellingandwellness.co.za/docs/TraditionalMedicinebriefing.pdf

Røkke, M. (2004). *Witch' Hunt in Contemporary Tanzania Exploring Cultural and Structural Factors Leading to Violence Against Women in a Sukuma Village.* University of Tromsø Faculty of Social Sciences. https://munin.uit.no/bitstream/handle/10037/6530/thesis.pdf?sequence=1&isAllowed=y

Royer, P. (2005). The spirit of competition: Wak in Burkina Faso. *American Anthropologist, 107*(2): 295–296.

Sandel, M. J. (2007). *The Case against Perfection: Ethics in the Age of Genetic Engineering.* Harvard University Press. Retrieved from: https://DOI10.1007/s10790-010-9202-8.

Schmidt, G. (2005*). Contemporary Beliefs about Witches and Witchcraft in Kenya.* African Culture. Retrieved from https://citeseerx.ist.psu.edu/viewdoc/download?doi=10.1.1.495.9299&rep=rep1&type=pdf

Stollznow, K. (2010). *Football Gazing: Sports and Superstitions in South Africa.* Retrieved from www.csicop.org/specialarticles/show/football_gazing_sports_and_superstitions_in_south_africa

Tebbe, N. (2007). Witchcraft and Statecraft: Liberal Democracy in Africa. *Georgetown Law Journal, 183* (2007), 185–236.

The Voice. (2012). Muti in Politics. Retrieved from www.thevoicebw.com2012/05/18/muti-in-politics/

WADA Code (2021). The 2021 Prohibited List. Retrieved from www.wada-ama.org

WADA Code (2022). The 2022 Prohibited List. Retrieved from: https://ita.sport/resource/2022-prohibited-list/#:~:text=The%202022%20Prohibited%20List%20is,are%20banned%20in%20particular%20sports

Welbourn, F. B. (1968). Atoms and Ancestors. Western Printing Services Ltd. Retrieved from https://people.ucalgary.ca/~nurelweb/books/atoms/fred.html

Westlund, D. (2006). *African Indigenous Religions and Disease Causation: From Spiritual Beingsto Living Humans.* Boston, MA: Brill Leiden. Retrieved from https://ebookcentral.proquest.com/lib/nottingham/reader.action?docID=3004158

Wheating, A. (2018). *The Complete Olympic Creed. High Performance West.* Retrieved from www.highperformancewest.com/blog/2018/5/30/the-complete-olympic-creed

Winkler, A. S., Mayer, M., Ombay, M., Mathias, B., Schmutzhard, E., and Jilek-Aall, L. (2010). Attitudes Towards African Traditional Medicine and Christian Spiritual Healing Regarding Treatment of Epilepsy in a Rural Community of Northern Tanzania. *African Journal of Traditional, Complementary, and Alternative Medicines, 7*(2): 162–170. Retrieved from: https://journals.athmsi.org/index.php/ajtcam/article/view/648/520

World Health Organization. (2008). *Traditional Medicine*. Retrieved from www.who.int/mediacentre/factsheets/fs134 /en/

Wyk, I. W. C. (2004). African Witchcraft in Theological Perspective. *HTS Theological Studies, 60*(3). Retrieved from www.researchgate.net/publication/45681366_African_witchcraft_in_theological_perspective

Chapter 11

"Dopogenic" Environment and Doping in African Sport

Beullah Matinhira

11.1 Introduction

The use of illegal drugs to enhance performance in sports, technically referred to as doping, remains a significant international issue. Research has blamed the "dopogenic" environment for initiating and perpetuating the use of performance-enhancing drugs (PEDs) in sports among athletes. This chapter concurs with the fact that, indeed, the "dopogenic" environment forms the solid basis for abusing PEDs by athletes. Doping is the technical term in sports for using prohibited substances to enhance performance. Athletes have used technology and science to improve their performances, including lightweight tennis racquets and biodynamic running shoes. However, this chapter restricts the scope of research to drug use-related sports enhancement since drug use has more devastating effects, primarily on athletes' health, than any other technological devices. As such, studying the role played by the "dopogenic" space in formulating an anti-doping strategy is a task that many researchers have not fully explored. This area has often been ignored, and more focus and blame have been shouldered on the individual athlete. Against this background, this chapter aims to fill this research gap by highlighting the nexus between various environmental factors and the use of PEDs in sports.

The rationale behind studying the "dopogenic" space is exposing the reality that sport-related drug abuse is not only an individual choice but exhibits the interconnectedness of human relationships. Hence, the "dopogenic" area is embedded in communality, reciprocity, and interrelatedness. These values providing fertile ground for sport-related drug abuse can be positively harnessed to formulate an anti-doping strategy in Africa. More importantly, this chapter aims to show how a critical analysis of the various factors that form the basis of African ethics can be used as lasting tools for the eradication of doping and also for the formation of solid human bonds, which will, in the long run, help in the war against drug abuse in sport. As such, analysing the "dopogenic" environment, which sums up the recognition and appreciation that doping is not caused by a single factor but a combination of factors, becomes relevant, especially for Africa.

DOI: 10.4324/9781003370796-13

11.2 The Dynamics of Drug-Related Doping

The use of PEDs in sport has been designated as a form of cheating, deemed unfair and incompatible with the spirit of sport. Yesalis and Bahrke (2002) argue that the use of PEDs has become rampant in sport because of the competitive nature of sport and lucrative financial rewards. The phenomenon has reached alarming levels as the effects are far reaching not only for the sporting fraternity but also for the public health in general. Doping comes in various forms. According to Lippi and Franchin (2008), doping is conventionally referred to as the use of forbidden drugs to enhance performance in sport and increase athletic advantages. Yesalis and Bahrke (2002) further point out that the last half of the nineteenth century saw the beginnings of modern medicine and a notable growth in the use of drugs and other substances to improve sport-related performance. They additionally note that this period also marked the beginning of scientific experimentation with the anabolic effects of hormones.

They further highlight the definition of doping by the World Anti-Doping Agency (WADA), which is worth noting. From the WADA definition I am going to make use of the sections which are the most relevant for this chapter. According to WADA as cited in Lippi and Franchin (2008, p. 3), doping is defined as (1) the presence of prohibited substances or its metabolites or markers in athletes' bodily specimen; (2) the use or attempted use of a prohibited substance; (3) the possession of prohibited substances and methods; (4) the trafficking of any prohibited substance; (5) the administration or attempted administration of a prohibited substance or a prohibited method to any athlete, or assisting, encouraging, aiding, covering up, or any other type of complicity involving an anti-doping rule violation or any attempted violation. The last part of the definition of doping clearly spells out the reality that doping is socially situated as various stakeholders can actively participate in causing an athlete to abuse drugs to enhance his/her performance.

11.3 Understanding Dopogenic Environment

The phrase "dopogenic environment" has been coined as a way to shift focus from blaming the individual for drug abuse in sport and recognise that the environment has a lion's share in promoting a conducive space for doping to take place. The study of the "dopogenic" environment takes into cognisance important factors that heavily influence doping to take place. Lippi and Franchin (2008) view doping as a complex and multifaceted phenomenon involving a number of causes and factors that do not originate in the athlete field alone. In most cases athletes alone have been blamed for abusing drugs to increase performance-suffered stigma and even expelled from the sporting arena. Yesalis and Bahrke (2002) share the same sentiment that the press, sport federations, politicians, and medical community have solely blamed the athlete for abusing drugs to enhance their performances. However, according to Lippi and Franchin (2008) the overriding motivations behind athletes' drug abuse include enhancing their performance, pressure for success, and the need to meet expectation of others. Backhouse et al. (2017) group the factors that contribute to the "dopogenic" environment into two, namely, the structural- and the local-level factors. They argue that the local factors in the form of team, sports clubs, neighbourhood, home, and school work hand in hand with the structural factors such as educational systems, societal attitudes, and national and international organisations to form a conducive doping environment.

In emphasising this view, Lippi and Franchin (2008)) argue that the phrase "dopogenic environment" has universality as its main feature, which appreciates the fact that it is made up of factors such as, but not limited to, societal norms and values, industry, marketing, media, drug policies, and anti-doping and the health care systems. Moreover, the term "dopogenic" designates the availability of plenty of resources. Backhouse et al. (2017) share the same sentiments that the dopogenic environment does not turn a blind eye to the totals of influences produced by the environment. Yesalis and Bahrke (2002 attributes doping behaviour by athletes to the desire to satisfy the public and this desire is esteemed higher than the health of the athletes. This explains the fact that athletes are given pressure by the environmental factors to engage in doping. Hence, the solution for doping should come from the consideration of a combination of factors.

Moran et al. (2008) extend the view that drug availability and the environment in which an athlete trains in are some of the important factors which most researchers have often neglected. They further claim that access to doping products, conducive training environment, team mates, and competitors, alleviating pain, the role of the coach, and economic and monetary considerations are some of the factors that make the doping space more favourable. These factors play a significant role in giving pressure not only to the individual players but also to the whole team, thereby leading to a systematic programme being put in place. This means that most of the athletes have little or no control over systematic doping.

For Moran et al. (2008), team work has a considerable share of causing doping among team mates who share common beliefs. The desire to fit in the society remains an integral part of the group. Even the coach might be one of the greatest agents of doping. The fact that banned drugs can be easily smuggled to the buyer shows indeed that the "dopogenic" environment is a web of factors entangled within each other. According to Yesalis and Barkhe (2002), trainers play an important role in initiating experiments with a variety of drugs and poisons. Researchers, educationists, medical experts, media personnel, sports administrators, and policymakers should basically have the same priority and goals as far as anti-doping is concerned. Indeed, the dopogenic debate does not rule out the role of the individual athlete in taking the responsibility for abusing drugs for the sake of enhancing performance.

Technological innovations have aided the use of PEDs in sports, thereby strengthening the bonds in the "dopogenic" space. Lippi and Franchin (2008) cite the availability of plenty of stores which offer a variety of doping products. Most of these stores are virtual and difficult to identify and to be policed. Lippi and Franchin(2008, p. 24) talk of the "dopogenic" environment as the World Wide Web which promotes the smuggling of doping drugs and substances through a networking system. This implies that technological innovation can push doping further underground and make some drugs more dangerous and undetectable, hence increasing the risk for athletes.

The medical fraternity has been viewed as one of the fields which provide a fertile ground for doping. When tracing the history of the use of drugs for enhancing performance in sport, Yesalis and Barhke (2002) share the view that medical communities participated in the development and selling of illegal drugs for sport-related purposes. They further argue that physicians and trainers played an active role in administering powerful stimulants.

The scientists and sport federation officials in the United States of America were responsible for the institutionalisation of the use of PEDs. Moreover, the coaches made these substances available and encouraged their use, while sport federations were covering up for doping. Yesalis and Bahrke (2002) completes the cycle of the dopogenic environment by explaining the role of the society in causing the athletes to abuse drugs in the name of sports. He contends that society emphasises rewards, speed, strength, size, aggression, and winning. There is no doubt that all these factors leave the athlete with no choice but to be pressurised into using PEDs in sports. Yesalis and Bahrke (2002) further comments that doping is demand driven as the fans will be demanding high-level performance from their athletes, which forces the athletes to do anything to satisfy the desires of their fans.

11.4 Adopting the "Dopogenic" Approach as a Lasting Anti-Doping Strategy

The "dopogenic" environment has been largely portrayed as a space that promotes the abuse of drugs for enhancing performance in sport. However, this section aims at showing that a critical analysis of the dopogenic environment can effectively help one in finding lasting ant-doping solutions. Backhouse et al. (2017) champion the adoption of the "dopogenic" approach to tackling doping through the implementation of more innovative and analytical approaches. According to Lippi and Franchin (2008), evidence has shown that the implementation of anti-doping awareness campaigns and the intensification of in- and out-of-competition testing have not deterred the doping behaviour. Research evidence shows that the implementation of anti-doping measures cannot be fully effective unless they are based on studying a combination of factors that contribute to doping. To address these research gaps, this section aims at analysing the role of multiple factors in enforcing anti-doping behaviours. Anti-doping strategies might not be effective unless the "dopogenic" space is analysed.

Considering that the "dopogenic" environment is applauding the role of the global effort to fight against sport's doping culture and to protect athletes from its negative effects. According to WADA (2015, p. 14),

> [T]he celebration of the human spirit, body and mind includes the following rules: ethics, fair play and honesty, health, excellence in performance, character and education, fun and joy, teamwork, dedication and commitment, respect for self and other participants, courage, community and solidarity.

This supports the central point of the "dopogenic" environment that focusing on the individual ignores the complexity of modern sport, where sport is taken as a business that involves the interconnectedness of more than one entity.

Adopting the "dopogenic" approach can therefore be the lasting solution for anti-doping. This approach offers a more holistic style where athletes' health will be catered for and the influence of competitive pressure is also taken into consideration. This approach to anti-doping will shift the blame, focus, and responsibility from the individual athlete to the "dopogenic" environment itself.

11.5 Education Campaigns: The Eyes of the Dopogenic Environment

Educational anti-doping programmes are some of the factors that should be taken into cognisance to ensure that studying the dopogenic environment would enable effective anti-doping strategies. Analysing the "dopogenic" environment is recognising that doping is not centred on the athlete alone but emanates from a combination of factors. Hence, people who are directly or indirectly involved in sporting activities are educated on the negative implication of doping, then loopholes, which may hinder the effectiveness of anti-doping strategies might be closed. Backhouse et.al (2017)acknowledges the importance of education in formulating an effective anti-doping strategy by giving four supporting points on the importance of education.

Specifically, it (a) encourages signatories to engage and leverage the resources and expertise of researchers and educational institutions, (b) stipulates that education programmes should be evidence-based and informed by educational theory and social science research, (c) requires signatories to seek partnerships with academics and members of research institutions to support evaluation and research, and (d) suggests that social science research should be used to inform evaluation procedures. Improving the uptake of research evidence into practice – by ensuring a greater degree of collaboration among researchers, policymakers, and practitioners – is critical to reducing the gap between research evidence and anti-doping decision-making.

Educational programmes are critical in enforcing the anti-doping ethical values in athletes and in any other stakeholder as well as closing the gap between research findings and anti-doping decision and policymaking. On the importance of educational programmes, Lippi and Franchin (2008) argue that there is a great need to ensure that ethical education and guidance for the athletes are of the highest standard. Snow (1999) supports the importance of educational campaigns in doping-related issues by stating that, "the International Standard for Education (ISE) reflects a growing recognition of the importance of education within the policies and practices of the organisations that form the global anti-doping community". Their use of the phrase "anti-doping community" implies that education is not important solely for the athlete but for various stakeholders as well.

The "dopogenic" space emphasises the importance of a community of persons who are ready to win the war on doping. Broadely (2021) further argues that anti-doping education is important because it discourages putting much emphasis on punishment as tertiary prevention but rather focuses on primary prevention. WADA as cited in Broadley (2021) stresses the point that education should be the top priority for all anti-doping programmes and athletes should get in contact with education before other doping testing measures.

Backhouse et al. (2017) argue that the shifting of focus from the individual athlete to the prevailing sporting environment contributes to an effective anti-doping strategy. According to Yesalis and Bahrke (2002, pp. 6–7),

> Although it has taken over a century there presently appears to be a consensus among various interest groups, including many athletes, physicians, coaches, administrators and spectators that performance enhancing drug use in most sports is a serious and growing problem.

More importantly, the dopogenic environment spells the spirit of sport which is the core rationale for anti-doping regulations.

11.6 Medical Personnel

Medical experts play a crucial role in the formulation of anti-doping policies and practices; they can also be responsible for drug-related research and administering of substance for sports enhancement. Hence, without looking into how they participate in the doping and anti-doping paradigm, the research will be deemed incomplete. Lippi and Franchin (2008) share the view that for anti-doping strategies to be effective general practitioners and sport physicians should play an active role. Backhouse et al. (2017, p. 6) support this view by calling the medical professionals to actively prescribe and promote evidence based on effective alternatives to doping. More importantly the sports physicians should focus more on forming partnerships to do doping-related research and challenge any practices that make the dopogenic environment thrive.

To really position the "dopogenic" environment into context, Backhouse et al. (2017) push for an idealised whole system of operationalisation of the "dopogenic approach" for the promotion of the interconnectedness of activities and structures in tackling the dopogenic environment. The same value of teamwork can also be used for the good cause of doping prevention. Lopez et al. (2010) argue that the medical profession has been one of the driving forces in reacting against doping. Dimeo (2007) adds that the zeal for anti-doping came from the medical staff who dealt with doping not only from a health perspective but also from a moral one.

11.7 The Role of Technology and Media in the Promotion of "Dopogenic" Approach to Anti-Doping

The world is technologically advancing on a daily basis. There is no doubt that technological advancement can cause doping to be more intensified, undetectable, and more harmful. Technological advancement has made it easier and faster to detect athletes who dope, but it has also helped make it easier to dope. However, many researchers have been made to believe that same technology can be harnessed to formulate a lasting anti-doping strategy within the context of the "dopogenic" environment. Pitassi and Leandro (2018) emphasise the need for increasingly advanced technologies in designing anti-doping solutions to match the existence of advanced doping techniques that resulted from technological revolution. For them doping is a biomedical technological issue that has to be addressed from the perspective of innovation theory. Lopez et al. (2010) also share the same view that "Performance enhancing techniques and substances should be primarily and precisely considered as a form of bio-medical technology".

In this section I argue that we cannot talk of the dopogenic environment in the twenty-first century without analysing the role of technology in formulating an anti-doping strategy. Of course, technological advancement has been used to modify doping and make it almost undetectable, but in this section, I am going to focus more on the positive role played by technological innovations in strengthening the "dopogenic" approach to anti-doping.

The use of PEDs in sport remains a contentious global issue that has become increasingly prevalent in the media over the years. The media has been blamed for fuelling the use of performance-enhancing substances in sport. Most of the media reports portray the success story of athletes as the only thing that should be cherished, hence triggering the passions of athletes to win at all cost. As such, there is no doubt that media players contribute immensely towards the development of anti-doping moral strategies.

There is no doubt that a close relationship exists between sport discipline and ethics. The relations are premised on the human interactions involved in sporting activities. Sporting activities also result in the formation of more human bonds. It becomes crystal clear that we cannot talk of sport without really taking the ethics discourse on board. The deontological nature of sport which manifests in the discipline being rule-based makes ethical in scope, suggesting also that solutions to the challenges faced in sport should be sought from ethical discourses. .

11.8 Conclusion

Though the "dopogenic" environment has been interpreted negatively to refer to a wide range of interconnected factors that provide a conducive environment for doping behaviour, I have argued that the careful scrutiny of the same phenomenon can be used as an anti-doping strategy. From the above discussion I have also demonstrated that indeed doping is a worldwide complex concern. The complexity of doping is made possible by the interconnectedness of various factors that complement each other. Doping is found in various forms, which range from blood to technological forms. However, this research was restricted to drug-related doping since it is one of the ancient forms of doping. I have demonstrated that ethical principles should be considered when dealing with doping issues in order to formulate an effective anti-doping strategy. I have therefore established that there is a need to harness a variety of factors, structures, organisations, individuals, and teams in the fight against doping other than just focusing on the individual athlete. It is my submission and recommendation that athletes, society, teams, coaches, media houses, medical experts, researchers, and other related personnel (the dopogenic environment) need to work and co-exist in the fight against doping, thereby formulating an effective anti-doping strategy.

References

Backhouse, S. H., Whitaker, L., and Petroczi, A. (2017). Gateway to Doping? Supplement Use in the Context of Preferred Competitive Situations, Doping Attitude, Beliefs, and Norms. *Scandinavian Journal of Medicine and Science in Sports, 23,* 244–252. https://doi.org/10.1080/19406940.2018.1528993

Broadley, B. C. (2021). *Anti-Doping Strategies in Sport*. New York: Rowman and Littlefield.

Dimeo, P. (2007). *A History of Drug Use in Sport 1876–1976: Beyond and Evil.* London and New York: Routledge.

Lippi, G., and Franchin, E. (2008). Doping in Competition or in Sport. *British Medical Bulletin, 9,* 235–316

Lopez, J. C., Ruiz, F. J., Feder, J., Barbero-Rubio, A., Suarez-Aguirre, J., Rodríguez, J. A., and Luciano, C. (2010). The Role of Experiential Avoidance in the Performance on a High Cognitive Demand Task. *International Journal of Psychology and Psychological Therapy, 10*, 475–488.

Moran, P., Desna, B., and Lacos, T. (2008). Preventing Doping in Sport: An Investigation of the Attitudes and Perceived Role of High Performance Coaches. Unpublished. Moran Project.

Pitassi, C., and Leandro, R. L. (2018). Technological Capability of Doping Control Laboratories: A Metric Proposal. *International Journal of Sport Policy and Politics, 8*, 18–37.

Snow, B. (1999). *Drug Information: A Guide to Current Resources*. 2nd ed. Lanham, MD: Scarecrow Press.

WADA (2015). International Standard for Testing and Investigations. *World Anti-Doping Agency*. Canada.

Yesalis, C. E., and Bahrke, M. S. (2002). History of Doping in Sport. *International Sports Studies, 24*(1), 267–278.

Chapter 12

Conceptualising *Juju* as a Form of Doping in the Malawian Soccerscape

Dave Mankhokwe Namusanya

12.1 Introduction

Doping has long been highlighted as unfavourable in sports because of its adverse effects on the health of athletes. Further, it also negatively impacts the spirit of sports, especially in reinforcing unfair advantage (Killowe and Mkandawire, 2005). Understanding of doping, however, has been chiefly scientific, with the world body responsible for promoting anti-doping practices – the World Anti-Doping Agency (WADA) – mainly relying on what are referred to as considerations of doping primarily driven by the physical evidence of doping (Kovač, 2016). This largely ignores other realms of unfair sports practices that are prevalent in usually non-Western societies such as Africa. This chapter reconsiders the conceptualisation of doping within Africa, particularly in Malawi.

The chapter builds on the narratives of *Juju* that blighted the Malawi National Football Team, the Flames, campaign at the Africa Cup of Nations (AFCON). This campaign highlights the perversity of *Juju* within the African social and public spaces. The focus is on the narratives of *Juju* that became a part of the campaign, which was labelled mainly a success by Malawian football lovers and commentators (see, for example, Muheya, 2022). In reflecting on these narratives, especially as they mirror and shape society's attitudes towards and knowledge of sports, the chapter also aims to add depth to the literature that has challenged conceptualisations of doping within African cultures. The argument that this chapter advances is inspired mainly by the work of Kovač (2016), who sought to contextualise the use of *Juju* within African football as own African views of doping. Thus, this chapter does not just present issues of *Juju* as realities within African football as other works have done (see, for example, Asamoah-Gyadu, 2015; Njororai, 2020; Schatzberg, 2006) or romanticising them as African traditional religion as the work of Chipande et al. (2019) did; instead, it situates the issues within the need to redefine doping, making it undoubtedly relevant to African societies.

In a way, one must think of the work in this chapter as a decolonial exercise. This chapter is a rejection of Western viewpoints as the gold standard.

DOI: 10.4324/9781003370796-14

It is a decentring of knowledge from the global northern hemisphere, deliberately equating it with expertise from the areas that have long been considered as the peripherals (Said, 1978). All this is done with the backdrop of the Flames' campaign at the AFCON.

When the Malawi National Football Team qualified for the 2021 AFCON finals in Cameroon, few people allowed them to proceed beyond the group stages. The refrain was the same in public places, on social media, and mainstream media: the Flames were going to the continental showpiece to register their presence. Indeed, a trawl through local newspapers and social media posts reveals people's low expectations of the team, with one columnist declaring that "expecting the Flames to perform wonders...is at one's peril" (Ndovi, 2022, para. 5). Companies and politicians, usually eager to associate themselves with successful brands, deserted the team, so it had to host golf tournaments to raise money for the competition (Chilemba, 2021). Indeed, the expectation was so low that when the team succumbed to a goal defeat in its first game of the tournament against Guinea, there was little complaint. In the next match, against Zimbabwe, Malawi's win became a national celebratory event, with the nation coming to a literal standstill. And when it held the eventual champions Senegal to a goalless draw in its last match before subsequently qualifying for the knock-out stages, the tale of triumph had been cemented. The narrative of the unbelievable finally happening had long been established, with one journalist declaring that Malawi had charmed the world with its performance (Muheya, 2022).

However, as this narrative of a justified success – or what Schatzberg (2006) would refer to as the scientific processes of football – run came another underneath it: the success of Malawi was nothing other than the work of *Juju* (Zvomuya, 2022). Thus, the fact that such a lowly regarded team had managed to go beyond its expected levels could only be attributed to the world of the supernatural. Of course, the allegations had been long running in the Malawian social space ever since images had been published of the Flames kit master boarding with the team on its journey to Morocco. This had, however, just been treated as light talk until the team started registering its success. Success can only be the work of *Juju*, thus says common knowledge in the African "soccerscape" – the word being taken from the work of Schatzberg (2006), who quoted sports sociologist Richard Giulianotti to refer to the social and political structures around football. *Juju* – or what would broadly be understood as magic, witchcraft, or sorcery – is not just a material reality within the African social space; it is integral to African sporting (Kovač, 2016; Pannenborg, 2008).

12.2 Methodology

In making its case on redefining doping, this chapter focuses on the Flames at the AFCON in Cameroon. Media reports of the journey, as well as reflections of the journey within the social imaginary, are the ones that are mostly relied on to reflect on the campaign. Here, the media is taken as a performative and actual space where human experiences, interactions, and realities are documented and presented (Reifsnyder, 2018). Narratives of *Juju* are therefore taken as a reflection of the epistemologies within the community (see, for example, Daimon, 2010, who has argued on violence in football as manifesting the grander picture of police–citizen relationships within society). Thus, the materials used in this chapter – lifted across different media platforms – are not just taken as carefully curated and sanitised realities. They are rather taken as reflections of the everyday life that is mirrored as well as subsequently shaped by the media. This, of course, is done mindful of the reality that in themselves the media outlets are places of power in which powerful entities reproduce what they deem as knowledge (see, for example, Mohammed, 2022). Power, however, is taken here to mean what is regarded as the norm within the context (Reifsnyder, 2018).

The media materials identified and subsequently used in this chapter were analysed using a content analysis technique. As per Hsieh and Shannon's (2005) argument, content analysis is especially relevant for text data as it allows for a subjective interpretation of the text. In this chapter, data constituted the printed words found in the texts that are being referred to, to drive the argument. As the chapter leans on the normalisation of *Juju* practices to highlight their visibility within the Malawian soccerscape, especially through media (Reifsnyder, 2018), the curated materials that have been used are mostly from newspaper reports and social media (particularly Twitter). Background information was sourced from newspaper (both print and online) reports, while the data under focus was obtained from reports and reactions on the Flames 2021 AFCON campaign. This was for social media posts made in January 2022 and a news reporter carried on New Frame, an online publication that focuses on African news.

12.3 Epistemological Viewpoint

A particular position on knowledge grounds this work. This is what I call an epistemological viewpoint. This viewpoint has been inspired by the work of various African and other non-Western scholars that have called for the decolonisation of knowledge in all its forms (Mohammed, 2022; Ndlovu-Gatsheni, 2015; wa Thiong'o, 1992; Said, 1978). The argument, as posited by such scholars as Ngugi wa Thiong'o (1992), is that the way of looking at the world is largely colonial, with knowledge of colonial masters privileged as the only way of understanding the world. People from the other worlds, such as Malawi in this case, are then taken in as subjects of that viewpoint with their own ways of understanding the world labelled as savage or uncivilised. Indeed, as Said (1978) pointed out, the Western viewpoint operates as a core of knowledge and other societies are regarded as the peripheral; in this peripheral, the people occupying such spaces cannot define their own realities. They are rather defined and categorised. Their knowledge, observed Santos (2016), is often dismissed as ignorance.

However, ways of understanding the world are multiple. Reality is often a product of social constructions that in themselves are not void of biases (Said, 1978). Indeed, each of the ways of knowing and looking at the world has its own advantages and disadvantages (Santos, 2016). It is this realisation of the multiplicity of knowledge and viewpoints that necessitates the need for a continuous evaluation of what is regarded as knowledge. This approach, subsequently, supports the need for decolonising knowledge. Knowledge, as Ndlovu-Gatsheni (2015) argued, needs not be only that accepted by the Western world as knowledge.

Boaventura de sousa Santos (2016) makes a perfect case for decolonising knowledge, arguing for what he calls an ecology of knowledge in which all knowledges are treated as equal and complementary. The argument is that at the limit of one knowledge, another comes to address such limits. In this position, no knowledge is central nor is there any other knowledge outright dismissed as ignorance or just mere fetish just because it cannot be conceptualised within the scientific realm. In contextualising the epistemological position within the arguments of this chapter, it should be noted that no knowledge of doping is central and certainly more important to be regarded as the absolute while its very existence seeks to relegate other considerations of the same. In discussing unfair advantages over others in sport then, such knowledge from what the non-physical aspects of sport would be regulating much of life in non-Western societies should be considered (Daimon, 2010; Kovač, 2016). These are equally valid viewpoints. Their existence is a reality for millions of other people even if we find that reality disagreeable.

12.4 Redefining Doping in Africa

WADA has defined doping as the use of substances and/or methods that gives competitors an unfair advantage over others and enhances their performance (WADA, 2021). Doping agents, apart from giving unfair advantage, can also be harmful to the health of competitors (Killowe and Mkandawire, 2005). This certainly seems straightforward as long as the performance-enhancing substances are known, which constitute drugs that are oftentimes illegal. However, as Kovač (2016) has pointed out, in Africa there are also methods through which sports personalities as well as their supporters believe that performance can be enhanced and that those who use such methods get to have an unfair advantage over their competitors. Such a method is the use of magic or what is commonly known as *Juju* (Daimon, 2010; Pannenborg, 2008).

As argued by Njororai (2020) who echoes the observations of both Kovač (2016) and Asamoah-Gyadu (2015), issues of magic are quite common in African sport. Indeed, both spectators and sports personalities believe that for a win to happen in sport there has to be the use of some special powers. These special powers are what one would say are the ones that WADA finds unlawful and aims to tackle. However, as Kovač (2016) has advanced, in a reminisce of the seminal work of Evans-Pritchard (1937), the space in which this form of doping occurs is within the supernatural. That is, it is a practice that is far out of sight and sometimes happens long before the matches. It should nevertheless be highlighted that in a significant number of cases, some teams and sports personalities have been accused of the same in the course of sports activities (Schatzberg, 2006). In his reflection of the same practice of using *Juju* within football, Daimon (2010) has indicated how some *Juju* practices entail that players will spend the night at the graveyard. Thus, to prove this would be hard although it is the case that such events indeed happen and are regarded as effective by the people who practise them. In Malawi, for instance, there have been reports of disruptions in football matches over activities that the other teams have long held as indicative of *Juju* – or to quote the language of this chapter "doping". Malenga (2017), for instance, reported that one renowned football supporter had declared that all the football in Malawi's elite league is under the influence of *Juju* (much of this is discussed in the next section). The research by Killowe and Mkandawire (2005) also revealed that at least 70% of football players in Malawi believed that *Juju* influences football success.

The challenge, however, with accepting *Juju* as a form of doping is that its substance effects are not well known. Indeed, as Kovač (2016) has highlighted, most of the *Juju* practices in African football are not just about what one takes; rather, they are mostly about things that one can bath in, tuck in sport paraphernalia, and even what they can just believe. They are, so to quote Schatzberg (2006), "difficult to investigate" (p. 353). Where success is achieved after *Juju* practices, the scientific community refers to it as a case of chance (see, for example, Daimon, 2010; Schatzberg, 2006). However, as recorded from WADA's own conceptualisation of doping, it is not just about the use of particular materials to enhance performance that would pass for doping, it is also in the use of some other methods that seek to give the user an unfair advantage (WADA, 2021). This, therefore, makes issues of *Juju* interesting as far as doping is concerned. Evans-Pritchard's (1937) argument that magic and witchcraft are not an objective reality, yet a reality for the people who hold the belief remains true. As Kovač (2016) highlights, in African societies it is the case that the spiritual non-objective world is always in constant co-existence with the physical world. Similar views have been advanced by Asamoah-Gyadu (2015) and Chipande et al. (2019) albeit from a Christian religious perspective where African traditional religions are mirrored as relative to Christianity.

What emerges from the foregoing, nevertheless, is that to successfully define doping within the African context means broadening the WADA (2021) conceptualisation of doping. It is to borrow much from decolonial literature and conversations and decentre Western notions that seek to separate the body from the mind or the physical from the spiritual. From the arguments advanced by such scholars as de Sousa Santos (2016) as well as Mohammed (2022), it is to acknowledge that the world cannot only be viewed from monolithically adjusted lens; rather, the world can be viewed from different and varying standpoints. Indeed, in most parts of such countries as Malawi, it is hard to find the chemicals that are used for doping, yet in the common experiences of sport, *Juju* practices continue to dominate and the practice is held strongly by both players and officials alike (Malenga, 2017; Killowe and Mkandawire, 2005; Ndovi, 2017b).

While critics might challenge that it would be hard to intervene in spiritual aspects of the issue and indeed advance that issues of *Juju* cannot be equated with doping, it is important to point out that there have been scenarios where football authorities in Africa have had to step up and punish teams as well as individuals that have done practices which have long been associated with *Juju* tendencies (Ndovi, 2017a; Schatzberg, 2006). Thus, the point here is that acknowledging the practice, and regarding it as one of doping, creates ways through which societies and associations that believe – or indeed operate in such contexts that believe – in the practice can get to address it, especially considering the impact that such practices have on sports development (this is discussed in detail in Section 12.7).

12.5 Doping and *Juju* in Malawi

The allegations against the Malawi National Football Team that it had travelled with it a *Juju* man were not new in the Malawian soccerscape. Football in Malawi has long been shrouded in this spiritual realm of *Juju* that the media has also picked up on such issues with interactions ranging from reporting incidences of suspected *Juju* use (Malenga, 2017), creating narratives of *Juju* use (Ndovi, 2017a), and, to a lesser extent, outright dismissal of such issues (Mlanjira, 2017). Those who dismiss such issues usually rely on the arguments that *Juju* does not work or, if it did, then the teams using it would have had been successful (see Zvomuya, 2022). However, to dismiss such issues just because of their perceived unworkability is to ignore the larger context in which they operate and would even be argued to be a neo-colonial attitude towards knowledge, which this chapter seeks to challenge and undo.

In order to discussing *Juju* within the Malawi soccerscape, significant focus should be on the elite league: the Super League where in 2017 it was reported that at least 2 million Malawi Kwacha (about U$2500 at the time) was spent by each team in a match on *Juju* practices which were termed as "research" (Ndovi, 2017b). This points to an impact of this practice on Malawian football: depriving resources from the areas that need them, such as player welfare which, by all standards, is poor in Malawi. Furthermore, as it was recorded in the same report, *Juju* practices were also destroying sports infrastructure, with the teams involved needing to plant their substances on the football pitch. A similar tactic of planting substances on the football pitch was also recorded in Cameroon by Pannenborg (2008). These might have an impact on the sports infrastructure, with heavy costs on sports development. This is yet another way that *Juju* practices seek to redefine doping. The practices do not only have an impact just on the teams using them, they also have an impact on the broader sports development (Kovač, 2016).

Thus, it might not be completely remiss to argue as Mlanjira (2017) does that *Juju* is one of the factors hindering sports development in Malawi. The only umbrage one can take from his argument is to dismiss the workability and, therefore, the validity of *Juju* beliefs. This, as already highlighted, is a neo-colonial position in which the knowledge of other societies is regarded within the measure set by Western approaches (Thiong'o, 1992). It should, however, be clearly highlighted that the situation of football in Malawi is quite complex that one factor is not enough to be accused of having such a huge impact on sports development. Indeed, what is accepted is that like what is taken as doping in the other world that relies on chemical substances, *Juju* has even similar impacts on sports development, personalities as well as their welfare, and the facilities that they have to use. This, therefore, does not only make *Juju*'s use highly controversial (Schatzberg, 2006), but also necessitates the need to consider within the academia as well as find ways of addressing it in general sports management.

12.6 Transcending the National Stage: The Flames and *Juju* Allegations

The narratives of *Juju* in the Flames campaign did not just start with their success at the AFCON. They have always been pervasive, with a 2015 news report having quoted the Chief Executive Officer of the Football Association of Malawi at the time confessing that the team uses *Juju* (Khamula, 2015). It was with such a background that when the team, in 2021, released pictures of their journey to Cameroon via Saudi Arabia, the reports were back to haunt them. As a photo of the squad circulated, attention was focused on the team's kit manager, hitherto little known, whom people alleged was the team's *Juju* man and was bound to help the Flames deliver miracles in Cameroon.

In its first match where it suffered a defeat, not much was said about the *Juju* man as the team had performed to expectations or – to situate it within the context of this chapter – no "African doping" had been used. It was, however, when the team defeated Zimbabwe and held the eventual champions, Senegal, to a goalless draw that the rumours gained momentum. As companies back in Malawi were outsmarting each other by making donations and promises to the team, on social and mainstream media the rumours started running rife: Malawi had a *Juju* man. It was mostly the amplification of the rumour by Malawian social commentator, with a wider reach on social media, Idriss Nassah, that the rumour grew legs. In a Tweet, he posted a photo of the kit manager with a caption suggesting that the person was not a "kit manager"; rather, he was a "*Juju* man".

His Tweet gained ground, with over 300 reTweets, as he attracted a flurry of comments in which some equally laughed with him (the Tweet had an emoji at the end to indicate light talk) while some admonished him. The storm, nevertheless, had started. The rumour had gained a footing such that it was across Africa with Zimbabwe – mostly doing it out of the malice of its own loss at the hands of the Flames – running far along with this rumour. As a Zimbabwean also posted on Twitter after the same match: Malawi must have been doing *Juju*.

To the question of why Zimbabwe would not have unleashed its own *Juju* operations, the response was provided by a Zimbabwean journalist, Percy Zvomoya (2022): the Malawi team would just have had a better *Juju* man or the contest was not just worth it for Zimbabwe *Juju* men since Malawi is renowned for its *Juju* prowess.

From that moment, Malawi's success came to be tied to *Juju*. In their match with Senegal, there was little talk of *Juju*. For all practical purposes, the match had not lived to its expectations. It was, however, in the knockout match against Morocco that the rumours came again. Malawi had taken a lead within the first 7 minutes of the match and for a better part of the first half, they appeared to fend off the constant attacks of the Moroccan side. This again triggered the allegations of *Juju* on the social media space. Social commentators, shocked by the resilience, had not to look farther than the Flames and Malawi's record in *Juju* for explanation.

A user, however, in what can be termed as the stretching of the definition of doping wondered if there was a way of ascertaining that a team was using *Juju*. The way Morocco was missing chances could only be expressed as the work of *Juju*. Thus, they posted that "They (perhaps meaning CAF or FIFA) should configure VAR to detect *Juju* or voodoo. There is some weird stuff I am seeing in this Morocco match".

In the end, of course, Malawi lost the match. However, with a 76% possession for Morocco against the Malawi National Football Team's 24% and a total of 24 shots on goal for the former against 4 for the latter, the 2 to 1 margin with which Morocco won the match was hardly an actual reflection of the match. Indeed, with that the reputation of Flames using *Juju* at the AFCON campaign as inquired by the news report of Zvomuya (2022) was only cemented.

12.7 Discussion

The general agreeableness of this *Juju* rumour, not only in Africa but specifically in Malawi, revealed how pervasive the *Juju* culture is. Its scaling to continental heights just highlighted how much within Africa *Juju* is regarded

(Zvomuya, 2022). Certainly, to label this as a non-issue simply because it is something that our systems have not yet devised ways of managing is a disservice. Indeed, a rhetorical question response to the one that Mlanjira poses in his opinion piece of why the Flames has not won the World Cup if *Juju* really works, one needs not go further than read through Pannenborg's (2008) work where this question was already answered by Africans who have long been dogged by this question: "European teams such as Germany and England simply have more modern and stronger forms of magic at their disposal" (p. 11).

Indeed, in rephrasing the same questioning tactic within the remits of this discussion, the question of doping cannot simply be dismissed because the users of unfair chemicals and methods have lost. It might be because the winners also used way more advanced methods than those who lost. Thus, the question of doping is not settled just by, and on, the outcome. It is settled rather by the consideration of the doping practices within their own context. In this chapter, the position advanced has been that there is a need to reconsider doping so that it considers other world knowledges long kicked to the curb by the interests of colonialism and capitalism that strive to present knowledge as monolithic – only as that which is within the physical world. The spiritual world, as Kovač (2016) argues, is conveniently disregarded. A reconceptualisation needs to bring into focus the spiritual world as well.

Redefining doping should not be considered just as an academic exercise. It is not just about creating a platform through which other knowledges can get their own space (wa Thiong'o, 1992) despite its importance. However, the point is that beyond the violence of erasure that ignoring such conceptualisations have on sports development, there is also an economic violence that such knowledges perpetuate. Failing to address such conceptualisations, therefore, makes sport less of a rewarding venture.

As previously highlighted, *Juju* practices were highlighted to have an economic impact on Malawian football. This was even true for the Flames AFCON tournament where the team was technically shunned by business which has long looked at it as a non-viable venture. Indeed, when the pictures of the so-called *Juju* man appeared with him joining the squad, people questioned the extravagance of the team considering that it was sailing in financial difficulties. It is these perceptions of *Juju*, and its attendant costs, that mask the reality of the nature of funding that Malawian football has, thereby casting the inadequacies rather as the lack of financial prudence and failures of the footballing authorities (Daimon, 2010).

12.8 Conclusion

The question of *Juju* having a place in African football is long gone. It might be wished away, pretended against or even dismissed as having no impact, yet the reality is that it happens and has significant bearing on sport practices within Africa broadly, and Malawi specifically. This chapter, however, aimed to broaden this conversation by not only focusing on scenes and narratives of *Juju*, but also situating them within the context of doping. In tracing the soccerscape in Malawi, especially in the public discourse, and tying it to the Malawi National Football Team, this chapter has advanced the need to consider *Juju* as a form of doping within African football. This is mostly regarded within its impacts on sportsmanship. *Juju* practices in themselves harm the development of sports. Thus, regarding them as harmless or an African obsession with no impact on football does a disservice to the development of African sport. Also, as other forms of *Juju* use include the ingestion of substances, it is important that there is focus on these not only as giving unfair advantages to the users, but also as harmful to the users.

References

Asamoah-Gyadu, J. K. (2015). "Christianity and Sports: Religious Functionaries and Charismatic Prophets in Ghana Soccer". *Studies in World Christianity, 21*(3), 239–259. https://doi.org/10.3366/swc.2015.0126

Chilemba, E. (2021, October 3). "Flames Fundraising Golf Tournament Rakes in K73.4 Million". *Malawi 24*. https://malawi24.com/2021/10/03/flames-fundraising-golf-tournament-rakes-in-k73-4-million/

Chipande, H. D., Mwale, N., & Chita, J. (2019). "Religiosity in African Football: 'Magic' and Christianity in the Zambian Game in Colonial and Modern Times". In C. Onwumechili (Ed.), *Africa's Elite Football* (pp. 238–251). New York: Routledge.

Daimon, A. (2010). "The Most Beautiful Game or the Most Gender Violent Sport? Exploring the Interface between Soccer, Gender and Violence in Zimbabwe". In J. Shehu (Ed.), *Gender, Sport and Development in Africa: Cross-cultural Perspectives on Patterns of Representations and Marginalization* (pp. 1–12). Dakar: CODESRIA.

Evans-Pritchard, E. E. (1937). *Witchcraft, Oracles and Magic among the Azande (Vol. 12)*. Oxford: Clarendon Press.

Hsieh, H. F., & Shannon, S. E. (2005). "Three Approaches to Qualitative Content Analysis". *Qualitative Health Research, 15*(9), 1277–1288.

Khamula, O. (2015, November 18). *FA Malawi CEO admits using Juju for national team*—Malawi Nyasa Times—News from Malawi about Malawi. Nyasatimes. www.nyasatimes.com/fa-malawi-ceo-admits-using-juju-for-national-team/

Killowe, C., & Mkandawire, N. (2005). "Knowledge, Attitude, and Skills Regarding Sports Medicine among Football Players and Team Doctors in the Football Super League in Malawi". *Malawi Medical Journal: The Journal of Medical Association of Malawi, 17*(1), 9–11.

Kovač, U. (2016, October 28). *'Juju' and 'jars': How African athletes challenge Western notions of doping. The Conversation*. http://theconversation.com/juju-and-jars-how-african-athletes-challenge-western-notions-of-doping-67567

Malenga, B. (2017, June 13). "Malawian Football Teams Use Juju". *Malawi 24*. https://malawi24.com/2017/06/13/malawian-football-teams-use-juju/

Mlanjira, D. (2017, May 31). "If Juju Works, Why Malawi Are Not World Champions?" – *Malawi Nyasa Times* – News from Malawi about Malawi [News]. Nyasatimes. www.nyasatimes.com/juju-works-malawi-not-world-champions/

Mohammed, W. F. (2022). "Bilchiinsi Philosophy: Decolonizing Methodologies in Media Studies". *Review of Communication, 22*(1), 7–24. https://doi.org/10.1080/15358593.2021.2024870

Muheya, G. (2022). January 26). "Malawi: Flames Charm the World After AFCON Sensation". *Nyasa Times*. https://allafrica.com/stories/202201260648.html

Ndlovu-Gatsheni, S. J. (2015). "Decoloniality as the Future of Africa". *History Compass, 13*(10), 485–496. https://doi.org/10.1111/hic3.12264

Ndovi, J. (2017a, May 31). "4 Teams Fined for Juju Rituals". *The Nation Online*. www.mwnation.com/4-teams-fined-for-juju-rituals/

Ndovi, J. (2017b, October 31). "Clubs Spend K2m on Juju, BNS Complains on Practice". *The Nation Online*. www.mwnation.com/clubs-spend-k2m-juju-bns-complains-practice/

Ndovi, J. (2022, January 9). Go Flames Go! *Nation on Sunday*, 10.

Njororai, W. W. S. (2020). "Culture of Magic and Sorcery in African Football". In C. Onwumechili (Ed.), *Africa's Elite Football* (pp. 99–116). New York: Routledge.

Pannenborg, A. (2008). *How to Win a Football Match in Cameroon: An Anthropological Study of Africa's Most Popular Sport*. Leiden: African Studies Centre.

Reifsnyder, L. (2018). *Jocks for Justice: How Sports Media Reflects and Propagates Societal Narratives* [CMC Senior Theses, Claremont McKenna College]. https://scholarship.claremont.edu/cmc_theses/1810

Said, E. (1978). *Orientalism: Western Concepts of the Orient*. New York: Pantheon.

Santos, B. de S. (2016). *Epistemologies of the South: Justice Against Epistemicide*. New York: Routledge.

Schatzberg, M. G. (2006). "Soccer, Science, and Sorcery: Causation and African Football". *Africa Spectrum, 41*(3), 351–369.

Thiong'o, N. wa. (1992). *Decolonising the Mind: The Politics of Language in African Literature*. Nairobi: East African Publishers.

Zvomuya, P. (2022, January 28). *Is That A 'Juju' Man on Malawi's Bench?* New Frame. www.newframe.com/is-that-a-juju-man-on-malawis-bench/

Chapter 13

African Sociocultural Context and WADA's Whereabouts Requirements

Manuel Kasulu, Stella Patience Mikwana, Agatha Magombo, and Yamikani Ndasauka

13.1 Introduction

This chapter assesses the efficiency and practicality of the World Anti-Doping Agency's (WADA) whereabouts requirements in relation to the African athlete. It argues that the whereabouts requirements are inconsistent with the communitarian nature and the two-dimensional conception of time predominant among Africans. WADA established the whereabouts requirements to combat out-of-competition doping among athletes. These whereabouts requirements demand athletes to provide their whereabouts information to enable anti-doping officials to locate them for unannounced testing during out-of-competition periods. This chapter proposes a modification of the current whereabouts requirements, which involves the introduction of geolocalisation as a replacement for the current whereabouts requirements to achieve WADA's objective of testing athletes during out-of-competition periods and to accommodate the sociocultural context of African athletes. The chapter is divided into five sections. The first section provides an introduction, the second section discusses the experience of the African athlete, the third section describes the communitarian nature of African communities, the fourth section analyses the challenges that African athletes encounter because of the structure of WADA's whereabouts requirements, and the fifth section offers a critical reconstruction of WADA's whereabouts system.

13.2 WADA's Whereabouts Requirements

Doping in sports is unethical and undermines the discipline's core values, such as fair competition among athletes (Henne, 2010, p. 307). Therefore, WADA, international anti-doping organisations, and national anti-doping organisations (NADOs) were established to uphold the integrity of sports and to eliminate practices of doping (Houlihan, 2014, p. 2; WADA, 2003). The anti-doping approaches adopted by WADA can be classified into two categories. The first category comprises procedures and measures, such as tests that WADA conducts during competitions, and the second category

DOI: 10.4324/9781003370796-15

includes the measures that WADA adopts to deal with doping during out-of-competition periods. The first category was WADA's primary and only approach to anti-doping until it was discovered that some athletes were using performance-enhancing drugs that retained their ability to improve performance during competitions but could not be detected during testing at the competitions. This discovery led to the adoption of the second approach, which was implemented to ensure that athletes were not using performance-enhancing methods outside of competition.

Therefore, the out-of-competition anti-doping strategy was crafted into a whereabouts system with requirements for athletes to provide their whereabouts information to anti-doping organisations throughout the year. WADA implemented its drafted whereabouts requirements in 2004 through the World Anti-Doping Code (MacGregor, 2013; Houlihan, 2014). These whereabouts requirements required athletes in the registered pool identified by international federations (IFs) and national anti-doping organisations (NADOs) to provide information about their home address, contact telephone numbers, future competitions, training venues, and travel plans to their respective anti-doping organisations (Waddington, 2010). In addition to providing this information, athletes were obligated to fill in their whereabouts information for each annual quarter on WADA's Anti-Doping Administration and Management System (ADAMS) software platform (MacGregor, 2013). Apart from storing the whereabouts data of athletes, the ADAMS platform also stores WADA's information such as anti-doping regulations which can be accessed by anti-doping organisations around the world and in so doing promotes efficiency, transparency, and effectiveness of anti-doping campaigns (Lapouble, 2017, p. 2).

The purpose of the whereabouts information was to make it possible for anti-doping officials to find athletes at their places of residence without any prior notice to the athletes. The rationale behind formulating the whereabouts strategy was to discourage athletes from engaging in doping practices even when they were not in competition because they could be tested at any time (Houlihan, 2014; Waddington & Møller, 2019). The whereabouts requirements were a reactive approach by WADA to the inadequacies of the existing in-competition testing procedures that were supposed to control doping practices in sports (Møller, 2011). Møller (2011, p. 178) further observes that the stand-alone in-competition testing measures were ineffective as athletes could easily circumvent them. For instance, athletes deliberately used prohibited drugs during out-of-competition periods that would be undetectable during in-competition testing but still have performance-enhancing effects during competitions (Møller, 2011).

The result of the intention to test athletes during out-of-competition periods was the need for anti-doping organisations to have information about the whereabouts of the athletes during these out-of-competition periods to efficiently fulfil their tasks (Borry et al., 2018). To ensure that athletes cooperated with the whereabouts requirements, WADA established sanctions accompanying the breach of the provisions. WADA also indicated that the missing of tests and filing failures would constitute an anti-doping violation, resulting in the suspension of athletes from the sport. The whereabouts requirements imposed more responsibility on athletes. The athletes understood that it was their obligation to ensure that they avoid any intake of prohibited substances and that they should make themselves available for testing during out-of-competition periods (Qvarfordt et al., 2021, p. 251; Gleaves and Christiansen, 2019).

However, WADA's whereabouts system was involved in controversies because of its lack of clarity on the punishments athletes who did not abide by the requirements were supposed to receive. In 2006, the UK Athletics Limited (UKA) suspended Christine Ohuruogu, a women's track athlete, for one year because of missing tests due to inaccurate reporting of her whereabouts. Ohuruogu appealed UKA's decision to the Court of Arbitration for Sport (CAS) (Halt, 2009, p. 271). Furthermore, the whereabouts requirements were criticised for not being clear on the meaning of a missed test, the number of missed tests, or filing failures that would constitute an anti-doping violation, and the whereabouts information that IFs and NADOs had to collect from athletes (MacGregor, 2013). MacGregor (2013) argues that the 2004 whereabouts requirements left these presented issues at the discretion of anti-doping organisations, which led to the criticism that the whereabouts requirements were unfair to athletes.

WADA addressed these concerns by revising the whereabouts requirements. In 2009, WADA implemented the newly drafted whereabouts requirements. WADA maintained most of the requirements, such as the provision for athletes to update their whereabouts information on ADAMS platform and give information about their contact details, home addresses, telephone numbers, training venues, future competitions, and travel plans to anti-doping authorities. Furthermore, WADA included a new provision for athletes to indicate to anti-doping authorities a one-hour slot each day between 6 am and 11 pm and a specific location for which anti-doping officials would find them for unannounced testing (WADA, 2009; Borry et al., 2018; Møller, 2011, p. 178). The revised whereabouts requirements require athletes to constantly update their whereabouts whenever they make changes on WADA's ADAMS software or through other means such as text messages or email as may be approved by WADA (Gleaves and Christiansen, 2019). WADA also emphasises that athletes can be sanctioned for failing to update changes in their whereabouts (Borry et al., 2018). In addition, the whereabouts requirements also indicate that anti-doping authorities can still test athletes outside the 6:00 hrs to 11:00 hrs time slot, but athletes would not be held to account if they miss this kind of test (Waddington, 2010). In the revised whereabouts requirements WADA explicitly indicates that three missed tests or failure filings within 18 months would constitute an anti-doping violation that would result in an athlete's suspension from the sport for one to two years (Borry et al., 2018). However, Borry et al. (2018) point out that the sanctions by WADA for offences of missed tests and filing failures are not automatic since athletes can avoid punishment if they can provide a convincing justification of their absence to the anti-doping organisation.

13.3 The African Athlete

African athletes struggle to perform well at international competitions compared to their counterparts from other parts of the world, such as Europe. Some of the reasons for their poor performances are lack of access to modern training facilities and limited time for preparation. It is noteworthy to point out that some athletes, particularly those from Kenya and Ethiopia, do extremely well at international running competitions. The success of these athletes has particularly been attributed to their genetic makeup (de Lira et al., 2014, p. 124). Most African athletes come from developing countries that do not have the financial capacity to provide their athletes with adequate and modern sports infrastructure. Luiz and Fadal (2011, p. 2) indicate that studies have demonstrated that the financial resources of a country are one of the most important indicators for the success of athletes who live in that country. Luiz and Fadal (2011, p. 2) show that countries such as the United States of America, Britain, and Australia usually have successful athletes because of the economic resources that these countries have and invest in sports. On the other hand, athletes like those from Africa usually have limited access to adequate and modern sports facilities and generally perform poorly at international competitions.

Numerous reasons indicate the uniqueness of the experience of the African athlete. This section advances an argument of the uniqueness of the experience of the African athlete that is grounded in two premises. The first premise is that the African athlete resides in a dominantly communitarian society, and the second one is that the African athlete subscribes to a unique conception of time. The idea that the African culture is communitarian has been supported by several scholars, which include Placide Tempels (1959), John Mbiti (1970), Ifeanyi Menkiti (1984), Kwasi Wiredu (1992), and Kwame Gyekye (1997). Most of the scholars that have articulated the communitarian nature of African societies have endorsed and built on Mbiti's (1970, p. 141) argument that the African's experience of existence can be summed up in the dictum – "I am because we are, and since we are, therefore I am". By this proposition, Mbiti (1970) emphasises the primary importance of the community in the face of the individual's existence. Mbiti's (1970) view is that Africans cannot exist outside of the community.

Mbiti (1970) further notes that, for Africans, the community takes precedence over the individual and that the community makes, creates, and produces the individual. In this sense, as Mbiti (1970) argues, the African owes their existence to the community. Mbiti (1970) also asserts that in African societies personhood is not something that an individual gets to possess for the mere fact that one is a human being, but rather it is something that an individual achieves through incorporation into the society. Menkiti (1984, p. 171) advances this view of incorporation, arguing that one cannot become a person in an African community without going through the long process of social and ritual transformation. Menkiti (1984) argues that an individual who has not been incorporated into society remains a mere dangler to whom the description of a person does not apply.

The views of Mbiti (1970) and Menkiti (1984) set out the experience of the African athlete as unique in comparison to the Western athlete. Both Mbiti (1970) and Menkiti (1984) present straightforwardly that in African communities the interests and values of the individual have a secondary status to that of the community. Menkiti (1984, p. 171) contends that in the traditional African view the "reality of the community takes ontological and epistemic precedence over the reality of individual life histories". This ontological and epistemic precedence that the community has over the individual implies that the individual has to tailor their actions and endeavours in a way that suits and supports the well-being and harmony of the community. Oyowe and Yurkivska (2014, p. 89) also argue that through the incorporation into the community, an individual is helped to understand and respect their obligations towards their immediate family and the community. At the root of these obligations is the principle that an individual has to put the harmony of the society first, which would mean that, at times, the individual would have to sacrifice their harmony for the balance of the community. Furthermore, Masolo (2010, p. 242) argues that the process of incorporation serves as a significant aspect of moral education in African societies. Masolo (2010) avers that through this moral education that is done through rituals and rites of passage, individuals acquire the values that help them live in ways that promote the community's social order.

The communitarian experience of the African is marked by a spirit of selflessness whereby individuals perceive themselves as simply a part of the whole community. Mbiti (1970) argues that when the African suffers, they do not suffer alone since they suffer together with the whole community. Again, when they rejoice, they rejoice with the entire community. Vivid examples of this solidarity in African societies can be observed during wedding and funeral ceremonies. During a wedding ceremony in traditional African communities, the community comes together and mobilises resources to support the couple getting married. The same happens during funeral ceremonies where the community mourns with the deceased's family. This sort of solidarity requires community members to leave their tasks for these kinds of traditions and put their resources at the service of the community. It is this solidarity in African communities that prompts Mbiti (1970, p. 141) to argue that whatever happens to the individual happens to the whole community.

Scholars such as Kwame Gyekye (1997) have objected to some ideas in the dominant conception of African communitarianism. Gyekye, advancing moderate communitarianism, has argued against Mbiti (1970) and Menkiti (1984) for presenting an extreme version of communitarianism that does not have a place for individual rights. Gyekye (1997) argues that despite individuals having obligations towards their communities, individuals in African societies also have individual rights that play a paramount role in their existence in the community. However, despite criticisms towards the conception of the communitarian nature of African communities, such as Gyekye's (1997), the views of Mbiti (1970) and Menkiti (1984) demonstrate that the centrality of the community in African thought is beyond contest. The dominant place of the community in African thought is also supported by Tempels (1959, p. 160), who argues that the African human being is a force influencing and being influenced by other forces. The idea that Tempels (1959) advances is that the African is a relational being that is inextricably bound in relations with the community.

The second premise that marks the experience of the African athlete unique is the African conception of time. One of the most significant analyses of the African conception of time is from Mbiti (1970). According to Mbiti (1970), time for the Africans means the composition of events that have occurred and those that are immediately to occur. As Mbiti (1970) elucidates, the implication is that the concept of time for the African does not include events in the distant future as part of the time. This means that to the Africans time consists of the past and the present. Mbiti (1970, p. 27) argues that in the African conception, "time is a two-dimensional phenomenon, with a long past, a present and virtually no future". Mbiti (1970) adds that it is for the reason that the events in the future have not been realised that Africans consider the future to be absent. He acknowledges that the African conception of time is different from the three-dimensional Western conception, consisting of an indefinite past, a present, and an infinite future. For Mbiti (1970), the Western conception of time is foreign to the African experience.

Mbiti's (1970) analysis of the African conception of time has significant implications. His presentation and conception of time suggest that it is unlikely for an African to plan for the distant future. In an experience of existence where an individual cannot practically consider the future as a constituent of time, it would be natural to imagine such an individual as one who, at best, can only afford to plan for the foreseeable future. In addition, it would be practically naïve to expect an African to keep to schedule for an ongoing task that goes far into the future. The analysis of Mbiti on the African conception of time helps us understand that the Western view of time as linear and proceeding infinitely into the future is overwhelmingly at odds with what the Africans conceive time to be. Mbiti argues that whereas time is thought to move forward in the Western understanding, in the African conceptualisation it moves backwards. The views of Mbiti on the African conception of time have also been supported by Kayange (2021). According to Kayange (2021), the analysis of the -li ontology in the Chewa language also reveals the existence of the two dimensions of time: the past and the present.

Of course, the two-dimensional conception of time has received some criticism. Gyeke (1978) and Mohatlane (2013) are two African scholars who have raised objections to the two-dimensional concept of time regarding how Africans look at time. Both Gyekye (1978) and Mohatlane (2013) suggest that Africans share the Western three-dimensional conception of time. However, this study observes that Gykye's (1978) and Mohatlane's (2013) arguments do not give a thorough and broad reflection of the African conception of time. Mbiti's (1970) conceptualisation of time is valid and represents Africans' dominant conception of time.

13.4 WADA's Whereabouts Requirements vis-à-vis the African Athlete

Two aspects set apart African athletes from athletes in other parts of the world: the communitarian society of which the African athlete is a part and the two-dimensional conception of time that the African athlete subscribes to. The following passages discuss the challenges of living in an African communitarian society and subscribing to the two-dimensional conception of time posing for the African athlete in maintaining their moral standing in the community and fulfilling their obligations to WADA by abiding by the whereabouts requirements.

WADA's whereabouts requirements expect athletes to fill in their whereabouts information for each prior annual quarter (Lapouble, 2017, p. 2; Gleaves and Christiansen, 2019). This requirement assumes that the athlete have complete control of their time to the extent that they can indicate the places they will be at every one of those days for the subsequent three months. In addition, this requirement assumes a considerable degree of predictability in the way the athletes live their day-to-day life, enabling the athletes to produce a schedule of how they expect to spend each day in the next three months. However, as Mbiti (1970) argues, the African athletes do not have their resources, let alone their time, to themselves. As members of the corporate group, the African athletes are obligated from time to time to use their time in the service of the community.

A typical example of an instance that demonstrates that Africans do not have full control of their time in their community is a funeral ceremony. Mbiti's (1970) argument that the whole community suffers when one member of the community suffers implies that when the death of an individual happens in the community, the community as a whole is expected to mourn with the bereaved family. In this case, it means that the African athletes who attend funeral ceremonies in different locations have, from time to time, to keep updating their whereabouts to WADA. It is thus unrealistic for the African athletes to keep updating their whereabouts accordingly for every unexpected event that requires them to be at the service of the community. Ultimately, the African athletes realise that they cannot abide by WADA's whereabouts requirements and fully fulfil their obligations to the community.

In addition, this study argues that apart from having challenges with managing their time, African athletes also face obstacles in acquiring and maintaining moral standing in their society because their obligations to sport are less likely to allow them sufficient time to pursue the community's moral educational process and to fulfil their responsibilities to the community necessary for them to obtain personhood. As Menkiti (1984) argues, in the African communitarian society, personhood is something that an individual can succeed or fail at. According to Menkiti (1984), a person must go through society's rituals and fulfil their obligations to their immediate family and community to succeed in personhood. Due to efforts to balance responsibilities to WADA and the community, an African athlete is likely to find himself outside the favour of the community. A case in point is WADA's requirement that athletes should be at a particular location at a specific hour every day of the week by which anti-doping authorities can find them for unannounced testing (Møller, 2011). With this requirement, African athletes would be in a dilemma about what to do if the community unexpectedly requires their service at another place while observing this whereabouts requirement.

In conflicting situations, African athletes would be in a dilemma of either pursuing their obligations as athletes or pursuing their commitments to the community as persons. The African athletes find themselves in this difficult situation because of the structure of the whereabouts rules that fail to consider the African athlete's sociocultural context. For example, Masolo (2004) and Manzini (2018) argue that in African communitarian societies, the community's good outweighs the individual's good. As such, the individual should be willing to sacrifice their interests for the harmony of society. With this entrenched belief in the supremacy of the community's values over the individual's values, it would not be practical to expect African athletes to strike a balance between their obligations to sport and their duties to the community.

The second aspect that also puts the African athletes in a problematic situation insofar as their obligation to WADA's whereabouts rules is concerned is the continent's conception of time. According to Mbiti (1970), Africans have a two-dimensional conception of time. Mbiti (1970) argues that time to Africans consists of a long past and the present. As pointed out previously, Mbiti (1970) maintains that the idea of a three-dimensional conception of time is foreign to the Africans. In fact, he clarifies that the African conception of time is different from the Western conception of time. WADA's whereabouts rule that requires athletes to fill in their whereabouts information before every quarter of the year is founded on the Western conception of time where the future constitutes an actual dimension of time. However, as Mbiti argues, the end is virtually absent in the African conception of time. It can be drawn from

Mbiti's argument that the two-dimensional conception of time limits African athletes from coming up and sticking to a schedule that spans for several months into the future. This discrepancy in the conception of the reality of time in the experience of an African athlete and the practical requirement to fill in one's whereabouts information three months in advance puts the athlete at a disadvantage in abiding by WADA's whereabouts rules.

13.5 Reconsidering WADA's Whereabouts Requirements

In light of the challenges that the current WADA's whereabouts system poses for the African athlete, this chapter proposes a reconstruction of WADA's approach to out-of-competition testing. This reconstruction is founded on the values of personal freedom and trust. The current whereabouts system denies athletes personal freedom and treats them as irresponsible individuals always seeking opportunities to use prohibited substances and hence must be under strict surveillance (Møller, 2011, p. 187). WADA can accomplish its objectives and improve its relationship with athletes by modifying its current whereabouts system by abolishing some requirements in the current whereabouts system and introducing geolocalisation. Some of the conditions that may have to be repealed include the need for athletes to spend one hour at one particular location each day waiting for a possible unannounced test, athletes indicating specific areas of their whereabouts to WADA each quarter, and the rule that three missed tests in the space of three months are equivalent to a doping violation. In addition, a restructured whereabouts system would require athletes to report to WADA once each quarter stating the area they will be residing in that period and that the athletes would only update anti-doping officials if their whereabouts have changed. In this case, WADA will know the area in which a particular athlete is, and geolocalisation can be used if WADA wishes to identify the actual location of the athlete. Again, bearing in mind that different athletes may have other preferences on the exact type of geolocation technology instrument/device to use, this chapter proposes that WADA should approve a range of tools and devices that athletes can choose from depending on their value systems.

Furthermore, since technological progress is constantly increasing, WADA should include a deliberate policy in its reformed anti-doping framework that regularly reviews its out-of-competition testing approach. This periodic review would assess the challenges and opportunities the employed geolocation devices offer and recommend improvements wherever needed through deliberations with athletes. In the following passages, this chapter demonstrates that geolocalisation has numerous advantages for the African athlete and has already been identified as a welcome approach by athletes.

The approach of geolocalisation of athletes using location-based devices instead of the current whereabouts requirements has already received tremendous support from several athletes worldwide (Borry et al., 2018, p. 456). In fact, due to the demands from athletes and several other concerned parties for WADA to consider geolocalisation as a possible approach to achieving out-of-competition testing, WADA's Ethics Panel discussed this matter in its 2016 meeting in Montreal and 2017 meeting in Lausanne (Borry et al., 2018, p. 456). However, in both conferences, WADA's Ethics Panel maintained that tracking technology presents serious ethical and data security challenges, so geolocalisation could not be recommended (Borry et al., 2018). Therefore, in the following passages, this chapter justifies why geolocalisation appropriately fits the sociocultural context of the African athlete.

Due to the obligations that African communities bestow on individuals, it is difficult for the African athletes to have meaningful control of their time to observe WADA's whereabouts requirements strictly. However, with the use of a smartphone that can help in the geolocalisation of the athlete or a tracking bracelet, the African athletes can have the freedom to meet their obligations to the community, such as attending rituals and ceremonies without worrying about missing a test. In addition, the African athletes can be sure that if anti-doping officials needed them for a no-advance-notice out-of-competition testing, they would track and find them at their present location.

The tracking technology also relieves the African athletes from having to fill in and continuously update changes of their whereabouts on WADA's ADAMS platform. According to Borry et al. (2018, p. 456), geolocalisation gives athletes the liberty from the laborious task of providing their whereabouts information to anti-doping authorities. Again, with the tracking technology, the African athletes will not have to face challenges in delivering their detailed whereabouts for every prior annual quarter. Furthermore, this will solve the African athlete's challenges of planning future remote events due to the unique two-dimensional conception of time dominant among Africans.

Geolocalisation of athletes for no-advance-notice out-of-competition testing presents opportunities that also extend to anti-doping authorities. According to Borry et al. (2018, p. 457), the geolocalisation of athletes would help anti-doping officials improve the interpretation of the data integrated into the Athlete Biological Passport (ABP). The ABP contains records of biomarkers such as haemoglobin, haematocrit, and red cell counts that implicitly portray the effects of an athlete's doping over time. These biomarkers are known to be affected by age, sports discipline, gender, ethnic origin, and altitude. However, the current testing method does not consider the altitude, which poses serious concerns for the accuracy of the interpretation of the data in the ABP (Borry et al., 2018, p. 457). According to Borry et al. (2018), global positioning system (GPS) technology would help anti-doping officials quickly get information about altitude and enhance interpreting of the data recorded in the ABP.

The introduction of geolocalisation for African athletes can also tremendously improve the relationship between anti-doping authorities and African athletes. According to McGregor (2013, p. 256), the current whereabouts system that requires athletes to regularly fill in their whereabouts information has been heavily criticised by athletes worldwide. In addition, Borry et al. (2018, p. 456) argue that athletes have expressed their discontent, sometimes through the courts, with the surveillance character of WADA's whereabouts system, its infringement of privacy, and the high costs and burdens it puts on athletes. Møller (2011) also presents more concerns that athletes have raised against the current whereabouts requirements. According to Møller (2011, p. 178), currently, athletes have to accept rigorous surveillance in reporting any plan or change of plan and suffer the torture of stress at the thought that their career would be ruined for a mere lapse of memory that can result in a missed test. Furthermore, Møller (2011, p. 179) stresses that the current whereabouts system is founded on WADA's mistrust of athletes and treats athletes as individuals who cannot be responsible. According to Møller (2011, p. 178), the mistrust attitude embedded within the current whereabouts rules fosters demoralisation among athletes. In the face of this seemingly unhealthy relationship between athletes and anti-doping officials, the adoption of tracking technologies can restore the trust and sense of respect that athletes should have towards WADA and its establishment that seek to promote the interests of the sport and those who participate in it.

Tracking technologies can have risks such as ethical and data security challenges, as the WADA Ethics Panel has maintained in its resolutions (Borry et al., 2018; Valkenburg et al. 2014). In addition, GPS technology and location identifying devices can affect the planning of anti-doping authorities since they only provide the present locations of athletes (Borry et al., 2018, p. 458). However, concerning the sociocultural context of the African athlete, geolocalisation employed as a complement to the proposed modified whereabouts requirements presents a better option when compared with the current whereabouts system. With this proposed approach, WADA can still afford to make unannounced testing on athletes during out-of-competition periods and, in so doing, achieve the original aim of the no-advance-notice out-of-competition testing. In addition, this proposed approach ensures the individual freedom of an athlete since the tracking technology is easy to manipulate and can be tailored to the interests of African athletes who can prefer to have a tracking application on the phone, wear a trackable bracelet, have an implantable chip, or have something modified that is in line with their values and beliefs.

13.6 Conclusion

In conclusion, while the current whereabouts system assists WADA in fulfilling its objective of testing athletes during out-of-competition periods, it comes at a cost as, at the same time, it severely injures the value system of an African athlete due to its inconsistency with the African sociocultural context. As demonstrated previously, the current whereabouts requirements conflict with the communitarian nature of African societies and the African two-dimensional conception of time. Therefore, this chapter has proposed restructuring WADA's current whereabouts system by reforming current requirements and introducing geolocalisation. This proposal considers geolocalisation a compliment, not an alternative to WADA's whereabouts system. Through this reconstruction of WADA's whereabouts system, the African athletes will have the opportunity to flourish both in sport and in their community and WADA, on the other hand, will be better equipped to combat anti-doping during out-of-competition periods.

References

Borry, P., Caulfield, T., Estivill, X., Loland, S., McNamee, M., & Knoppers, B. M. (2018). "Geolocalisation of Athletes for Out-of-Competition Drug Testing: Ethical Considerations. Position Statement by the WADA Ethics Panel". *British Journal of Sports Medicine, 52*(7), 456–459. https://doi.org/10.1136/bjsports-2017-098299

de Lira, C. A. B., Vancini, R., Fachina, R., Montagner, P., Pesquero, J., Andrade, M., & Borin, J. (2014). "Genetic Aspects of Athletic Performance: The African Runners' Phenomenon". *Open Access Journal of Sports Medicine, 5,* 123–127. https://doi.org/10.2147/OAJSM.S61361

Gleaves, J., & Christiansen, A. V. (2019). "Athletes' Perspectives on WADA and the Code: A Review and Analysis". *International Journal of Sport Policy and Politics, 11*(2), 341–353. https://doi.org/10.1080/19406940.2019.1577901

Gyekye, K. (1978). "The Akan Concept of a Person". *International Philosophical Quarterly, 18*(3), 277–287 https://doi.org/10.5840/ipq197818329

Gyekye, K. (1997). *Tradition and Modernity: Philosophical Reflections on the African Experience.* Oxford University Press.

Halt, J. (2009). Where Is the Privacy in WADA's 'Whereabouts' Rule?s *Marquette Sports Law Review, 20,* 25.

Henne, K. (2010). "WADA, the Promises of Law and the Landscapes of Anti-Doping Regulation". *PoLAR: Political and Legal Anthropology Review, 33*(2), 306–325. https://doi.org/10.1111/j.1555-2934.2010.01116.x

Houlihan, B. (2014). "Achieving Compliance in International Anti-Doping Policy: An Analysis of the 2009 World Anti-Doping Code". *Sport Management Review, 17*(3), 265–276. https://doi.org/10.1016/j.smr.2013.10.002

Kayange, G. M. (2021). *The Question of Being in Western and African Analytic Metaphysics: Comparative Metaphysics Using the Analytic Framework* (Vol. 438). Springer International Publishing. https://doi.org/10.1007/978-3-030-69645-0

Lapouble, J. (2017). "Athlete Whereabouts in the Context of the Fight Against Doping in Africa; Mission: Impossible?" *HAL (Le Centre Pour La Communication Scientifique Directe)*. https://hal.archives-ouvertes.fr/hal-02535898/document

MacGregor, O., Griffith, R., Ruggiu, D., & McNamee, M. (2013). "Anti-Doping, Purported Rights to Privacy and WADA's Whereabouts Requirements: A Legal Analysis". *FairPlay: Revista De Filosofia, Ética Y Derecho Del Deporte, 1*(2), 13–38. https://his.diva-portal.org/smash/get/diva2:660702/FULLTEXT01.pdf

Manuel Luiz, J., & Fadal, R. (2011). "An Economic Analysis of Sports Performance in Africa". *International Journal of Social Economics, 38*(10), 869–883. https://doi.org/10.1108/03068291111170415

Manzini, N. Z. (2018). Menkiti's normative communitarian conception of personhood as gendered, ableist and anti-queer. *South African Journal of Philosophy, 37*(1), 18–33. https://doi.org/10.1080/02580136.2017.1405510

Masolo, D. A. (2004). *Western and African Communitarianism: A Comparison*. In K. Wiredu (ed.), *A Companion to African Philosophy* (pp. 483–498). Blackwell.

Masolo, D. A. (2010). *Self and Community in a Changing World*. Indiana University Press.

Mbiti, J. S. (1970). *African Religions and Philosophy*. Doubleday.

Menkiti, I. A. (1984). "Person and Community in African Traditional Thought". *African Philosophy: An Introduction, 3*, 171–182.

Mohatlane, E. J. (2013). "Reflections of Mbiti's African Temporal Categories in Moshoeshoe LeBaruti (Moshesh and the Missionaries)". *Journal of Communication, 4*(2), 71–78. https://doi.org/10.1080/0976691X.2013.11884809

Møller, V. (2011). "One Step Too Far — About WADA's Whereabouts Rule". *International Journal of Sport Policy and Politics, 3*(2), 177–190. https://doi.org/10.1080/19406940.2011.579145

Oyowe, O. A., & Yurkivska, O. (2014). Can a communitarian concept of African personhood be both relational and gender-neutral?. *South African Journal of Philosophy, 33*(1), 85–99.

Qvarfordt, A., Ahmadi, N., Bäckström, Å., & Hoff, D. (2021). "Limitations and Duties: Elite Athletes' Perceptions of Compliance with Anti-Doping Rules". *Sport in Society, 24*(4), 551–570.

Tempels, P. (1959). *Bantu philosophy*. Présence Africaine.

Valkenburg, D., De Hon, O., & Van Hilvoorde, I. (2014). "Doping Control, Providing Whereabouts and the Importance of Privacy for Elite Athletes". *International Journal of Drug Policy, 25*(2), 212–218. https://doi.org/10.1016/j.drugpo.2013.12.013

WADA. (2003). *World Anti-Doping Code*. WADA.

WADA. (2009). *International Standard Testing*. WADA.

Waddington, I. (2010). "Surveillance and Control in Sport: A Sociologist Looks at the WADA Whereabouts System". *International Journal of Sport Policy and Politics, 2*(3), 255–274. https://doi.org/10.1080/19406940.2010.507210

Waddington, I., & Møller, V. (2019). "WADA at Twenty: Old Problems and Old Thinking?" *International Journal of Sport Policy and Politics, 11*(2), 219–231. https://doi.org/10.1080/19406940.2019.1581645

Wiredu, K. (1992). *Person and community: Ghanaian philosophical studies I* (Vol. 1). CRVP.

Chapter 14

Responsibility Gaps in Anti-Doping Initiatives in Malawi

Yamikani Ndasauka, Maya Kateka, Fiskani Kondowe, Simon Mathias Makwinja, and Akuzike Kafwamba

14.1 Introduction

The central role of athlete support personnel (ASP) in doping and anti-doping in sports has been a point of debate for decades now (Smith & Stewart, 2008). According to the World Anti-Doping Agency (WADA), an ASP is "any coach, trainer, manager, agent, team staff, official, medical, paramedical personnel, the parent or any other person working with, treating or assisting an athlete participating in or preparing for sports competition" (WADA, 2009, p. 128). There are different proposals for advancing this role historically, theoretically, and empirically. ASP play a critical role in managing doping and anti-doping. One of the roles of ASP is to provide anti-doping data, training, and awareness to their respective athletes. Despite the crucial role of promoting clean sports, there has been minimal research on attitude, understanding, and perception of their roles as ASP in promoting clean sports (Petróczi & Aidman, 2009).

Doping or using performance-enhancing substances is detrimental to athletes, sports, and society. Therefore, one primary purpose of WADA is to harmonise anti-doping efforts, including providing anti-doping education. WADA was created to promote, coordinate, and monitor the fight against drugs in sports. It is responsible for the World Anti-Doping Code, which has been adopted by more than 700 sports organisations, including international sports federations, national anti-doping organisations (NADOs), the International Olympic Committee, and the International Paralympic Committee. Its principal activities include scientific research, education, the development of anti-doping capacities, and monitoring the World Anti-Doping Code. The World Anti-Doping Code is a document that harmonises anti-doping policies, rules, and regulations within sports organisations and among public authorities to protect athletes' fundamental rights to participate in doping-free sports. The code covers prohibited substances, testing and investigations, laboratories, Therapeutic Use Exemptions, privacy and personal information protection, code compliance by signatories, education, and results management. As an umbrella organisation, WADA delegates work in individual countries to

DOI: 10.4324/9781003370796-16

regional anti-doping organisations (RADOs) and NADOs and mandates that these organisations comply with the World Anti-Doping Code.

The duties of RADOs are to coordinate and manage delegated areas of their national anti-doping programmes, which may include adopting and implementing anti-doping rules, planning and collecting samples, managing results, reviewing TUEs, conducting hearings, and coordinating education programmes at a regional level. There are five RADOs, one of which is the AFRICA Zone VI RADO, of which Malawi is a member. However, these duties cannot be achieved without National Anti-Doping Organisations (NADOs). NADOs form the first point of contact as local ASP. They are responsible for daily managing anti-doping initiatives at the country level. They are also responsible for the promotion and popularisation of these anti-doping initiatives (Kamber, 2011).

According to article 7.2 of the WADA international anti-doping education standard, NADOs are responsible for implementing and monitoring anti-doping education programmes in their respective countries (WADA, 2021b). Furthermore, article 7.2.1 of the International Anti-Doping Education Standard states that each NADO shall be the authority on education related to clean sport within their respective country (WADA, 2021b). NADOs should support the principle that an athlete's first experience with anti-doping should be through education rather than through doping control. Furthermore, WADA (2021a) indicated that NADOs are responsible for promoting anti-doping education, including requiring national federations to conduct anti-doping education in coordination with the applicable NADO.

Regardless of this responsibility bestowed on NADOs, Gatterer et al. (2020) indicated that the most common barriers to implementing doping prevention programmes reported by the NADOs were a lack of resources and difficulties in collaborating with sports organisations. The study recorded and evaluated doping prevention approaches through information and educational activities of NADOs and assessed the extent to which a multifaceted doping prevention approach was realised (Gatterer et al., 2020). The study concluded that there were inconsistencies between NADOs' self-report data and the implementation assessment and that possible explanations for this discrepancy might be found in the reported barriers.

Despite the challenges NADOs indicate regarding implementing anti-doping education to athletes and coaches, it does not translate to the NADOs' ceasing responsibility for anti-doping education. Article 7.2.2 of the International Anti-Doping Education Standard (WADA, 2021b, p. 15) states that:

> each National Anti-Doping Organization shall devise an Education Program for those under their authority and in their Education Pool. National Anti-Doping Organizations shall document an Education Plan to demonstrate how their Education Program will be implemented and

monitored. National Anti-Doping Organizations shall evaluate their Education Programs annually.

The second critical ASP are coaches. Coaches are responsible for positively influencing the athletes they work with by teaching them ethical behaviours and assisting them to excel using their natural abilities (WADA ADEL, 2018). According to WADA, clean sport means coaches are also up to date and in sync with their athletes' sports experiences, including the vulnerable moments. Simultaneously, it also means supporting their athletes through anti-doping experiences and counselling and advising athletes on anti-doping matters as mandated by the WADA Code (WADA ADEL, 2018). To achieve this, WADA suggests that coaches must take the opportunity to be educated on anti-doping matters through their NADOs.

In the same quest to ensure anti-doping education for coaches, WADA developed a Coach's Tool Kit in 2007 to assist stakeholders in facilitating a face-to-face anti-doping education workshop for coaches. In 2010, WADA translated the tool kit into two online services and launched them as CoachTrue Elite and CoachTrue Recreational (WADA, 2010). Regardless of this introduction, it did not limit NADOs from designing their anti-doping education programmes for coaches. For example, in 2012, UK Anti-Doping (UKAD) introduced Coach Clean, which like CoachTrue offers an online programme that utilises interactive scenarios to improve coaches' understanding of what anti-doping means for them and their sportspeople (UKAD, 2012). However, these anti-doping education provisions vary between national and international organisations.

Schon (1983), in his theory of reflection, posits that framing practitioners' roles determine the issues identified as "problematic" and the strategies developed to address them. In this regard, coaches who do not view anti-doping as part of their role would be less likely to identify potential issues surrounding athlete doping (Allen et al., 2013). On the other hand, they may unintentionally reinforce doping behaviour through their "inaction". On the contrary, coaches who see anti-doping as crucial to their role may recognise issues/situations that may predispose or tempt athletes to engage in doping behaviour (Allen et al., 2013). In addition to the aforementioned, research has demonstrated that coaches' perceptions of their coaching role guide their behaviours and the issues identified and acted on (Bennie & O'Connor, 2010; Gilbert & Trudel, 2001; 2004; Nash, Sproule, & Horton, 2008). Schempp et al. (2006) have argued that, regularly, experts tend to reflect upon their beliefs about their role to monitor their professional practices; thus, just like Schon's notion of reflective practice, these coaches may act to intervene and reduce the likelihood of athlete doping behaviour (Allen et al., 2013).

The third critical ASP are team doctors. Some physicians facilitated subtle artificial performance enhancement within a controlled anti-doping framework in the past. From the 1958 case of John Bosley Ziegler (team physician of US weightlifters) to the 2015 case of Grigori Rodschenkow (head of the WADA Anti-Doping Laboratory in Moscow), the role of physicians in facilitating the use of prohibited substances has been recorded in history (WADA, 2016). A study by Dikic et al. (2013) found that some sports physicians were unaware of the nuances of doping regulations and, most importantly, the list of prohibited substances. Moreover, several team doctors have been shown to have exercised poor judgement in doping matters, resulting in athletes being punished for doping offences based on doctors' negligence. In such circumstances, the failure of ASP jeopardises athletes' rights. Korn and Volker (2013) revealed a multi-layered contractual relationship between sports teams, physicians, hospitals, and sports associations, providing a string of incentives for doctors to support performance-enhancing drugs.

WADA developed the Sports Physician Tool Kit (2014) to share knowledge about doping and anti-doping issues with sports physicians. The toolkit also spells out the responsibilities of a sports physician to stay up-to-date with the latest doping regulations and avoid contributing to inadvertent doping. In addition, sports physicians are also responsible for creating a doping-free sports environment, as the athlete's health is paramount to the physician.

According to a study by Allen et al. (2013), a robust anti-doping foundation and role frame components such as clarity of responsibility, the potential for performance benefit, and the prevalence of testing also contributed to anti-doping having a low priority for many ASP. A study by Patterson and Backhouse (2018) shows that anti-doping organisations' ability to devise, implement, and evaluate anti-doping education programmes for coaches is hindered by a lack of resources, limited interagency coordination, and challenges to overcome negative perceptions of anti-doping efforts. The study further shows that policy expectations concerning anti-doping education for ASP are not fully operationalised. However, this could change if anti-doping education is made a key priority for decision-makers in sports organisations; hence, it is highly likely to also become a central priority for ASP (Patterson and Backhouse, 2018).

The WADA Code states that athletes are liable for banned substances in their bodies and outlines that they are expected to know and abide by the anti-doping rules, policies, and practices. Furthermore, WADA also provides the Anti-Doping Rights Act, which promotes athlete rights within anti-doping and ensures that they are clearly outlined, accessible, and universally applicable (UKAD, 2012). The Anti-Doping Rights Act states that athletes have the right to receive anti-doping education and information from anti-doping organisations, which corresponds with code article 18 of the International Standard for Education (Athletes' Anti-Doping Rights Act, 2020). Departing from this, it can be argued that as much as athletes are responsible for promoting the clean sport, especially themselves, other parties are equally responsible for ensuring that this objective is met by providing anti-doping education.

So, this chapter assesses athletes' rating of the ASP role as a source of trusted information on anti-doping. Further, it investigates whether the ASP themselves understand their respective roles. Understanding who is responsible for promoting clean sports is vital for both the athlete and society in general. This assists in allocating blame when anti-doping is not being achieved and allocation of praise if things are right.

14.2 Methodology

A mixed method (qualitative and quantitative) approach was adopted in this study. Specifically, the study utilised Key Informant Interviews (KIIs), Focus Group Discussions (FGDs), and a survey. The qualitative and quantitative analysis results have been triangulated to provide an understanding of the identified determinants. KIIs were done with coaches and MADO officials. FGDs were conducted with student athletes. The survey targeted university student athletes and professional and semi-professional athletes from the following sporting categories: football, netball, and track athletics.

Data were collected from three cities of Malawi's Southern (Blantyre), Central (Lilongwe), and Northern (Mzuzu) regions. Interview guides and interviewer-administered questionnaires were used to collect qualitative and quantitative data. For the survey questionnaire, we adapted a questionnaire used in a similar study assessing doping attitudes and knowledge for Turkish athletes (Ozkan et al., 2020).

We used purposive sampling for KIIs and convenience sampling for FGDs and surveys. Six KIIs were conducted with coaches and officials from MADO in all three regions of Malawi. In addition, we conducted three FGDs, one in a university in each of the three target districts. Each FGD will comprise eight athletes. For the survey, 255 athletes out of the target of 280, which was based on a finite population of approximately 6,000 athletes – football (2,500, 41.7%), netball (1,500, 25%), track athletes (400, 6.67%), and university student athletes (1600, 26.6%) – was reached, representing a 91% response rate.

Data from KIIs and FGDs were first transcribed and translated into English. Then, the data were analysed using thematic analysis. Thematic analysis is a method of analysing qualitative data that is usually applied to a set of texts, such as interview transcripts. The researchers closely examined the data to identify common themes – topics, ideas, and patterns of meaning that come up repeatedly. This approach allowed the researchers to analyse the data in five broad steps: familiarisation, coding, generating, reviewing, and defining and naming themes. Survey data were entered, cleaned, and analysed using STATA version 17 software. Graphical and numerical summaries were used to describe the data. We calculated the proportions of athletes' source of doping information, trust in this information, and how these are distributed across various sporting categories and demographic factors, for example, gender and age. Inferential statistics were also explored to develop models explaining the role of multiple elements in doping practices.

Table 14.1 Basic demographics

Variable	*Sporting category – n (%)*					
	Football	*Netball*	*Track athletics*	*Boxing*	*Student athlete*	*Total*
Gender	76 (100)	0 (0	18 (75)	18 (67)	45 (75)	**157(62)**
Male	0 (0)	68(100)	6 (25)	9 (33)	15 (25)	**93 (38)**
Female						
Age	[24/15,33]	[24/15,40]	[25/15,40]	[20/15,32]	[22/18,30]	**[23/15,40]**
[Mean/Min, Max]	52 (68)	43 (63)	16 (67)	23 (85)	53 (88)	**187 (73)**
15–25 years	24 (32)	23 (34)	3 (13)	4 (15)	7 (12)	**61 (24)**
26–34 years	0 (0)	2 (3)	5 (21)	0 (0)	0 (0)	**7 (3)**
Over 34 years						
Education	1 (1)	0 (0)	0 (0)	0 (0)	0 (0)	**1 (0.5)**
None	1 (1)	0 (0)	4 (17)	11 (41)	0 (0)	**16 (6.5)**
Primary	64 (84)	54 (79)	18 (75)	15 (56)	0 (0)	**151 (59)**
Secondary	10 (13)	14 (21)	2 (8)	1 (4)	60 (100)	**87 (34)**
Tertiary						
Religion	67 (88)	65 (96)	20 (83)	21 (78)	55 (92)	**228 (89)**
Christian	9 (12)	3 (4)	4 (17)	6 (22)	5 (8)	**27 (11)**
Muslim						
District	23 (30)	28 (41)	12 (50)	8 (30)	26 (43)	**97 (38)**
Blantyre	53 (70)	33 (48)	6 (25)	9 (33)	27 (45)	**128 (50)**
Lilongwe	0 (0)	7 (10)	6 (25)	10 (37)	7 (12)	**30 (12)**
Mzuzu						
Total	**76 (30)**	**68 (27)**	**24 (9)**	**27 (11)**	**60(24)**	**255(100)**

The study was conducted with complete adherence to ethical standards expressed in the Declaration of Helsinki. Before the commencement of the study, relevant authorisation was sought from the University of Malawi Research Ethics Committee, Malawi National Sports Council, and different sports associations in Malawi. The study obtained written informed consent from participants. However, due to other challenges, participants who could not sign their consent forms were asked to use their fingerprints to give consent. Participants were notified that there was no monetary benefit in participating in the study. However, as the survey took place when most sporting functions were in recess, a modest transport refund of less than $3 was given to the participants. Each participant was assigned a participation number, and only the participant number appeared with their responses. No physical discomfort or psychological risks were anticipated from participating in this study. Nevertheless, participants were notified that they could skip or withdraw from the study if they felt uncomfortable with a question.

14.3 Results and Discussion

Demographic Details

According to Table 14.1, most of the athletes interviewed were male (62%) compared to females (38%). Although relatively more athletes were in the 15–25 years age group for all sporting categories, netball (2%) and track athletics (21%) had a few athletes over 34 years old. Almost all athletes (99.5%) had some form of education, and a majority had secondary education in football (84%), netball (79%), and track athletics (75%). The proportions of boxers with primary (41%) and secondary (56%) education were similar. Most respondents were Christians, with a slightly higher percentage of Muslims in track athletics (22%). Overall, more respondents were from Lilongwe (50%) compared to Blantyre (38) and Mzuzu (12%).

Responsibility for Communicating Anti-Doping

To gauge who athletes thought was responsible for communicating trusted information about anti-doping, we asked participants to mention their source of information on doping and anti-doping. Results are presented in Figure 14.1.

As shown in Figure 14.1, firstly, most respondents from netball, track athletics, boxing, and student athletes get information from their coaches. However, the coaches expressed reservations towards anti-doping information. They cited a lack of training and adequate anti-doping knowledge related to doping. "As coaches, we lack the requisite knowledge of doping and anti-doping. So, we don't know what to tell our players," KII Netball.

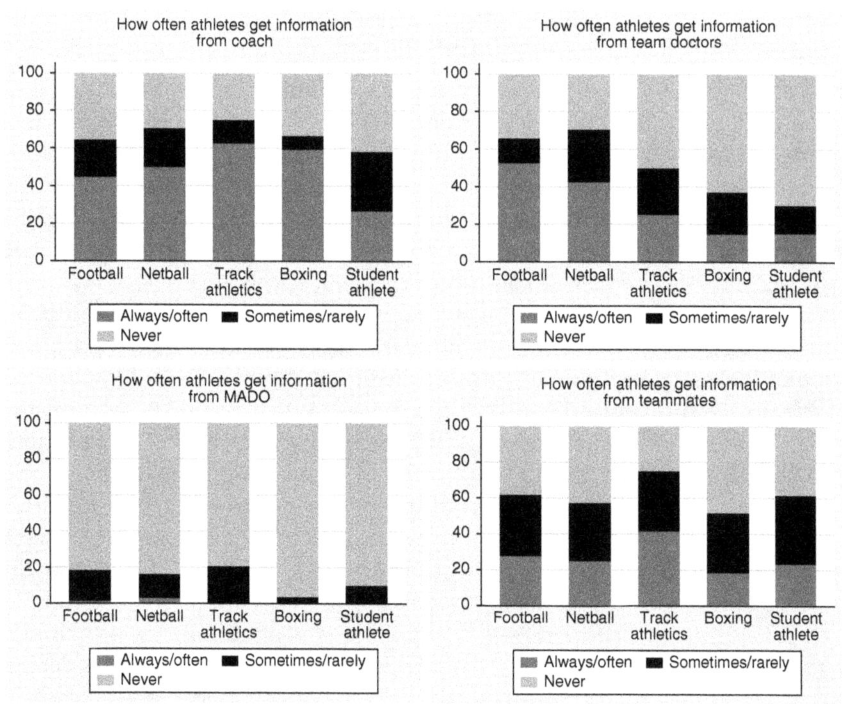

Figure 14.1 Participant's description of their sources of information on doping.

Secondly, athletes noted that they got information from team doctors and teammates. Ndasauka et al. (under review) found that 95% of athletes don't have adequate knowledge of doping and anti-doping in Malawi. This means that if teammates are the source of information, there is a chance that athletes don't pass on adequate information to their fellow athletes. Nevertheless, a study by Petroczi et al. (2021) revealed that doping or anti-doping is not a solo act. This means that team members play a significant role in promoting doping or clean sports. The historical influence of others, such as teammates, has already been acknowledged to play a role in instilling clean values and morals in athletes. Interactions with teammates create a bond of trust that would cause an otherwise clean athlete to inadvertently or intentionally dope (Petr'oczi et al., 2021). Further, Hughes (2013) notes that team doctors providing sports medicine services to high-performance teams often limit their involvement in illness and injury, allowing supplementation policies and protocols to be controlled by others in the organisation. Moreover, some sports physicians involved in positive doping cases are unaware of the nuances of doping regulations and, most importantly, the list of prohibited substances (Dikic et al. 2013).

Responsibilities for Enhancing Clean Sports

In the interviews, the participants mentioned the following institutions as responsible for promoting the anti-doping drive in Malawi: the Ministry of Sports, the Ministry of Health, the Football Association of Malawi, the Netball Association of Malawi, medical personnel, the Malawi Sports Council, and clubs. Although these institutions were mentioned, athletes did not think they, coaches, and other team officials are also responsible, except one who said that players are also responsible for clean sports. He said: "We players, team officials and coaches are responsible" (II Football). On the other hand, team doctors and coaches interviewed in the study expressed ignorance of their responsibility towards clean sports, citing a lack of knowledge of relevant information to enable them to carry out such duties. In a related study, Patterson and Backhouse (2018) found that coaches supported anti-doping efforts and exerted their influence by monitoring, giving advice, and creating the "right" culture. However, the coaches were reluctant to address anti-doping in their practice proactively, a situation exacerbated by a lack of self-efficacy to advise/act in accordance with the rules. Consequently, coaches tend to rely on others (both internally and externally to their club) to provide anti-doping support, and anti-doping is deemed unnecessary/irrelevant (Patterson and Backhouse, 2018). So, the hesitation of coaches and team physicians to lead in the anti-doping drive is not only applicable to Malawi. It seems to be a global phenomenon (see Backhouse & McKenna, 2012).

What is evident from the results is that athletes do not think that they are responsible for clean sports. Petroczi et al. (2021) showed that the clean athlete identity is generally rooted in upbringing, early experiences, and love of the sport. They are characterised by a continued, intrinsically motivated commitment to fundamental values and morals acquired in childhood. In contrast, clean performance enhancement is highly idiosyncratic and flexible. Furthermore, Petroczi et al. (2021) found that elite athletes recognise and value anti-doping efforts, but their experiences of disparity and unfairness in doping control undermine their trust in anti-doping. At the helm of the anti-doping strategy is the individual or collective athlete. The anti-doping drive becomes easier when athletes recognise their role in ensuring clean sports.

Surprisingly, MADO was conspicuously absent from the institutions that athletes mentioned as responsible for improving clean sports. Interviews with some sports associations and anti-doping organisations in Malawi revealed that most athletes do not know what doping or anti-doping is and do not have knowledge of the existence of an anti-doping body in Malawi. An official from the Netball Association of Malawi said, "athletes do not know about doping...when they hear the term doping, they just fear thinking they want to inject them or something...". Furthermore, the official expressed that they are unaware of anybody or any organisation that deals with issues of doping and anti-doping in Malawi. She said, "we lack doping experts to sensitise our athletes on the dangers of doping...we need to work together and form initiatives towards this fight against doping" (Netball KII 2).

Similarly, an official from the Athletics Association of Malawi (AAM) posited that because of a lack of knowledge, athletes and officials seem uninterested in the issues of doping and anti-doping. An officer from MADO echoed similar sentiments. He said, "yes, I remember that we tried to contact some officials from other sports associations. We have been trying to invite them for meetings or to fix some anti-doping awareness programs with them, but they have not been cooperating". He further posited that most associations do not appreciate the importance of MADO. However, MADO acknowledges that it is responsible for clean sports in Malawi alongside the Malawi National Sports Council, Malawi Olympic Committee, and the Ministry of Sports. In addition, the AAM official believes that responsibility falls in the hands of MADO and all leaders of sports associations in the country. In his statement, he says, "The responsibility of doping and anti-doping falls in the hands of MADO and all leaders of sports associations, but there is a need for constant reminders to athletes on doping and anti-doping education".

ASP play a crucial role in creating and fostering a clean sport culture that is not solely guarded by the threat of detection and sanctions. However, as is it clear from above there is a knowledge gap in understanding this role. The gap comes from various factors, including a lack of effective awareness programmes and enforcement of the existing guidelines. These problems were also noted in a study by Patterson, Backhouse, and Jones (2023), which revealed that there appeared to be ambiguity among other staff members regarding their anti-doping roles. The study also revealed that limited contact time, lack of knowledge, and the belief that a colleague is taking responsibility contributed to this gap in understanding respective roles. Similarly, Maznov et al. (2013) confirmed gaps in the knowledge of ASP, suggesting that more robust engagement with ASP anti-doping education and practice is needed.

14.4 Conclusion

This chapter investigated whether Malawian athletes, coaches, and MADO understand their role in promoting clean sports in Malawi. The results showed a discrepancy and systemic blame game between MADO and other sporting associations promoting clean sports in Malawi. This indicates a lack of clear strategy from MADO regarding implementing anti-doping programmes. By the power invested in them by WADA, it lies in their hands to ensure that athletes and coaches understand their roles in promoting clean sports. They are also responsible for mandating national associations to follow and carry out anti-doping education programmes. NADOs like MADO fulfil indispensable tasks in the national and international fight against doping. NADOs are the first "point of contact" for young athletes, their parents, and their national associations, where they receive their first information on doping prevention. Through the NADOs, they are notified about the damage doping causes to health and sportsmanship and their understanding of sports and sports ethics. Ensuring clean sports and playing true is everyone's responsibility. However, MADO is undeniably the supreme body entrusted with the commitment of the government and WADA to guarantee clean sport in Malawi. Regardless, the lack of a clear strategy to come up with critical responsibilities on clean sports among sporting bodies has negative implications on the work of MADO, especially the fight for a clean sport in the country.

References

Allen, J., Dimeo, P., Morris, R., Dixon, S., & Robinson, L. (2013). Precipitating or prohibiting factor? Examining coaches' perspectives of their role in doping and anti-doping. World Anti-Doping Agency. Social Science Research Scheme. *World Anti-Doping Agency Social Science Research Scheme*. www.wada-ama.org/en/Education-Awareness/Social-Science/Funded-Research-Projects

Backhouse, S., & McKenna, J. (2012). Reviewing coaches' knowledge, attitudes and beliefs regarding doping in sport. *International Journal of Sports Science and Coaching*, 6(1), 167175.

Bennie, A., & O'Connor, D. (2010). Coaching philosophies: Perceptions from professional cricket, rugby league and rugby union players and coaches in Australia. *International Journal of Sports Science & Coaching*, *5*(2), 309–320. https://doi.org/10.1260/1747-9541.5.2.309

Dikic, N., McNamee, M., Günter, H., Markovic, S. S., & Vajgic, B. (2013). Sports physicians, ethics and antidoping governance: Between assistance and negligence. *British Journal of Sports Medicine*, 47(11), 701–704. https://doi.org/10.1136/bjsports-2012-091838

Gatterer, K., Gumpenberger, M., Overbye, M., Streicher, B., Schobersberger, W., & Blank, C. (2020). An evaluation of prevention initiatives by 53 national anti-doping organisations: Achievements and limitations. *Journal of Sport and Health Science*, *9*(3), 228–239. https://doi.org/10.1016/j.jshs.2019.12.002

Gilbert, W., & Trudel, P. (2001). Learning to coach through experience: Reflection in model youth sports coaches. *Journal of Teaching in Physical Education*, *21*, 16–34. https://doi.org/10.1123/jtpe.21.1.16

Gilbert, W., & Trudel, P. (2004). The role of the coach: How model youth team sport coaches frame their roles. *The Sport Psychologist*, *18*, 21–43. https://doi.org/10.1123/tsp.18.1.21

Hughes, D. (2013). 'Organised crime and drugs in sport': Did they teach us about that in medical school? *British Journal of Sports Medicine* 47, 661–662. https://doi.org/10.1136/bjsports-2013-092570

Kamber, M. (2011). Development of the role of national anti-doping organisations in the fight against doping: From past to future. *Forensic Science International*, *213*(2011), 3–9.

Korn, E., & Robeck, V. (2013). The role of sports physicians in doping: A note on incentives. *MAGKS Joint Discussion Paper Series in Economics*, No. 17–2013,

Philipps-University Marburg, Faculty of Business Administration and Economics, Marburg.

Mazanov, J., Backhouse, S., Connor, J., Hemphill, D., & Quirk, F. (2013). Athlete support personnel and anti-doping: Knowledge, attitudes, and ethical stance. *Scandinavian Journal of Medicine & Science in Sports, 24*(5), 846–856. https://doi.org/10.1111/sms.12084

Nash, C. S., Sproule, J., & Horton, P. (2008). Sports coaches' perceived role frames and philosophies. *International Journal of Sports Science & Coaching, 3*(4), 539–554. https://doi.org/10.1260/174795408787186495

Ozkan, O., Torgutalp, S. S., Kara, O. S., Donmez, G., Demire, H., Karanfil, Y., et al. (2020). Doping knowledge and attitudes of Turkish athletes: A cross-sectional study. *Montenegrin Journal of Sports Science and Medicine, 9,* 49–55. https://doi.org/10.26773/mjssm.200307

Patterson, L. B., & Backhouse, S. H. (2018). "An important cog in the wheel", but not the driver: Coaches' perceptions of their role in doping prevention. *Psychology of Sport & Exercise, 37*(2018), 117–127.

Patterson, L. B., Backhouse, S. H., & Jones, Ben. (2023). The role of athlete support personnel in preventing doping: A qualitative study of a rugby union academy. *Qualitative Research in Sport, Exercise and Health, 15*(1), 70–88. https://doi.org/10.1080/2159676X.2022.2086166

Petróczi, A., & Aidman, E. (2009). Measuring explicit attitude toward doping: Review of the psychometric properties of the performance enhancement attitude scale. *Psychology of Sport and Exercise*, 3, 390–396. bhttp://dx.doi.org/10.1016/j.psychsport.2008.11.001

Petróczi, A., Heyes, A., Thrower, S. N., Martinelli, L. A., Backhouse, S. H., & Boardley, I. D. (2021). Understanding and building clean(er) sport together: Community-based participatory research with elite athletes and anti-doping organisations from five European countries. *Psychology of Sport & Exercise 55,* 101932.

Schempp, P. G., McCullick, B. A., Busch, C. A., Webster, C., & Mason, I. S. (2006). The self-monitoring of expert sports instructors. *International Journal of Sports Science & Coaching, 1*(1), 25–35. https://doi.org/10.1260/174795406776338490

Schon, D. A. (1983). *The Reflective Practitioner: How Professionals Think in Action.* New York: Basic Books.

Smith, A. C., & Stewart, B. (2008). Drug policy in sport: Hidden assumptions and inherent contradictions. *Drug and Alcohol Review*, 27(2), 123–129. https://doi.org/10.1080/09595230701829355

UK Anti-Doping. (2012). Annual Report and Accounts 2012/13. www.lawinsport.com/news/item/uk-anti-doping-publishes-annual-report-and-accounts-2012-13

WADA. (2009). World Anti-Doping Code. *World Anti-Doping Agency.*

WADA. (2010). CoachTrue Elite and CoachTrue Recreational. *World Anti-Doping Agency.*

WADA. (2016). McLaren Independent Investigation Report - Part I. *World Anti-Doping Agency.*

WADA. (2018). Anti-Doping Education and Learning platform (ADEL). World Anti-Doping Agency.

WADA. (2020). Athletes' Anti-Doping Rights Act. *World Anti-Doping Agency.*

WADA. (2021a). Code Review. *World Anti-Doping Agency.*

WADA. (2021b). International Standard for Education. *World Anti-Doping Agency.*

Chapter 15

Conclusion

What Now of Doping and Sports in Africa?

Yamikani Ndasauka and Simon Mathias Makwinja

15.1 Introduction

Doping in sports is a global issue that affects athletes from all regions, including Africa. Doping refers to using prohibited substances or methods to enhance athletic performance. These substances can include anabolic steroids, stimulants, hormones, and other performance-enhancing drugs. Athletics, particularly long-distance running, has been a sport where doping has been a significant concern in Africa. Countries like Kenya and Ethiopia, known for their success in distance running, have had cases of doping violations. The World Anti-Doping Agency (WADA) and other international bodies have closely monitored and tested athletes in these countries. Several factors contribute to doping in African sports. These include limited resources and infrastructure for anti-doping efforts, lack of education and awareness about the consequences of doping, financial pressures faced by athletes, and sometimes inadequate testing programmes. This book was particularly concerned about the theories and practices that inform doping in Africa, how athletes conceive of doping, and how they interact with WADA's rules, regulations, and policies.

15.2 The Practice of Doping in Sports in Africa

The origin of the word "doping" in Africa is still contentious. Some sources indicate that an African tribe, the Kaffirs, gave the name "dop" to a beverage that was consumed mainly in religious ceremonies as a stimulant drink (Conti, 2010). This clearly demonstrates that doping in sports is not alien to Africa. As Galafa (Chapter 3) demonstrates, the concept of doping can be viewed right from the imaginative thinking of Africans through such novels as *Kipjiru 42… 195*. In West Africa, athletes have been utilising the African plant *Catha edulis,* which contains pseudoephedrine, a psychomotor stimulant used to increase strength and delay the onset of fatigue (Ivy, 1983). From ancient times, West Africans used *Cola acuminita* and *Cola nitida* for running competitions (Boje, 1939).

DOI: 10.4324/9781003370796-17

What is distinct about the prevalence of doping in Africa is that athletes often refer to doping as *Juju*. As Mikwana et al. (Chapter 6), Mgungwe (Chapter 10), and Namusanya (Chapter 12) contend, the use of *Juju*, black magic, or witchcraft doping is relatively spread among athletes in Africa. *Juju*, "witchcraft", or "magic" are terms often associated with certain mystical cultural beliefs and practices in Africa. However, it is essential to note that the *Juju* concept varies across African countries and cultures. *Juju*'s association with sports is more of a cultural belief than a mainstream scientific proven phenomenon.

Nevertheless, the belief in *Juju* is prevalent among many Africans, more so among athletes. For example, in football (soccer), there have been reports of players or coaches using rituals or amulets believed to possess mystical powers to enhance their performance or weaken their opponents. Some players have been known to wear talismans or perform rituals before or during matches, believing it will bring them luck or protection. Spiritual doping in sports refers to using spiritual or religious practices to gain an unfair advantage over competitors. While spiritual doping is not commonly used in mainstream discussions on sports, it can be applied to situations where athletes rely on supernatural or mystical beliefs to enhance their performance.

Understanding that these beliefs and practices are not universally accepted or acknowledged in African sports is essential. Many people, including players, coaches, and administrators, do not attribute success or failure solely to *Juju* but rather to factors such as skill, preparation, teamwork, and luck. Nevertheless, Africa is diverse, with a rich tapestry of cultures and religions. Spiritual beliefs and practices vary significantly across different African countries and communities. Many African athletes, like athletes from other parts of the world, draw inspiration and motivation from their faith, rituals, or cultural practices. These beliefs and practices can provide a sense of confidence, focus, and mental fortitude, which may positively impact an athlete's performance. While spirituality and cultural practices can positively impact an athlete's mindset and performance, it is essential to ensure a level playing field in sports and adhere to established anti-doping regulations.

Assessing the extent or prevalence of spiritual doping in African sports is difficult, as it involves subjective and personal beliefs that may not be easily measurable or observable. Additionally, regulations and anti-doping policies in sports generally focus on performance-enhancing substances or methods that have a scientific basis and can be empirically tested. However, despite national anti-doping organisations' efforts to ensure clean sport in their respective nations, WADA needs to develop a position of *Juju*. This position must take into cognisance the view that *Juju* though not empirically verifiable is prevalent and dominates the discourse of doping in Africa.

Aside from *Juju*, another contentious issue concerns WADA's rules and requirements. This book has noted that applying WADA's rules is delineating, for they don't consider most of sub-Saharan Africa's cultural and economic context. Kasulu et al. (Chapter 13) demonstrate this vividly by analysing the

WADA whereabouts requirements. The authors argue that these requirements are inconsistent with the sociocultural context of African athletes and the two-dimensional conception of time that is predominant among Africans. African athletes live in predominantly communitarian societies with numerous obligations to their communities and immediate families. These obligations make it difficult for African athletes to abide by WADA's whereabouts requirements. The two-dimensional conception of time predominant among Africans also makes it challenging for African athletes to plan for future events. They hence propose a reconsideration of these rules. This is just one aspect that lacks proper cultural contextualisation of the rules of WADA.

15.3 Research on Doping in Sports in Africa

This is the first volume to consolidate interdisciplinary research in African anti-doping theory and practice. Nevertheless, there is a massive gap in research on anti-doping in Africa. This has been attributed to limited human capacity and research interest in doping. For instance, providing specific data on the prevalence of doping in African sports is challenging. Further, there is little interrogation of anti-doping policy and how athletes in Africa interact with these policies.

There is a need for more research into the prevalence of *Juju* as a form of doping or sports practice in Africa. Researching the psychological and physiological influence of *Juju* on athletes is also essential. Efforts to address doping in African sports are crucial to maintaining the integrity of competitions and protecting the health and well-being of athletes. Collaboration with international anti-doping organisations, ongoing education, and stringent testing protocols are essential to combatting doping effectively.

Lastly, research is needed regarding the anti-doping education framework in Africa. Education on doping in sports is crucial to effectively prevent and address the issue. One challenge faced in combating doping in African sports is inadequate education. Limited access to testing facilities, educational programmes, and awareness campaigns can contribute to doping-related issues. Specific research on best education practices about doping in sports in Africa is limited. This book shows that indigenous educational frameworks must be adapted to anti-doping initiatives. However, these frameworks should be adopted after assessing their efficacy.

15.4 Conclusion

African countries participate in international sporting events, such as the Olympic Games, World Championships, and continental tournaments. These competitions typically have anti-doping measures, including testing protocols and adherence to the WADA Code. While the belief in *Juju* and its association with sports exists in certain African cultures, it is not a universally accepted or recognised phenomenon. Most African sports rely on skill, training, and fair competition, just like in any other parts of the world. To combat doping, many African countries have established national anti-doping organisations and implemented anti-doping education programmes. These organisations work to educate athletes about the dangers and consequences of doping, promote clean sports, and conduct testing to detect the use of prohibited substances. International sports governing bodies, such as WADA, primarily focus on detecting and preventing substance-based doping rather than spiritual doping. However, if specific rituals or practices involve the use of banned substances or methods, they would fall under the jurisdiction of anti-doping regulations.

References

Boje, O. (1939). Doping. *Bulletin of the Health Organization of the League of Nations, 8*, 439–69.

Conti, A. A. (2010). Doping in sports in ancient and recent times. *Medicina nei Secoli, 22*(1–3), 181–190. PMID: 21560989.

Ivy, J. (1983). Amphetamines. In M. Williams (Ed.), *Ergogenic Aids in Sport* (pp. 101–127). Champaign, IL: Human Kinetics.

Index

Note: Page locators in **bold** and *italics* represents tables and figures, respectively.

For Product Safety Concerns and Information please contact our EU representative GPSR@taylorandfrancis.com
Taylor & Francis Verlag GmbH, Kaufingerstraße 24, 80331 München, Germany

www.ingramcontent.com/pod-product-compliance
Lightning Source LLC
Chambersburg PA
CBHW060302220326
41598CB00027B/4208

* 9 7 8 1 0 3 2 4 4 1 6 5 8 *